The Question of Competence

A VOLUME IN THE SERIES

The Culture and Politics of Health Care Work

edited by Suzanne Gordon and Sioban Nelson

A list of titles in this series is available at www.cornellpress.cornell.edu.

The Question of Competence

Reconsidering Medical Education in the Twenty-First Century

Edited by
Brian D. Hodges and Lorelei Lingard
with a Foreword by M. Brownell Anderson

ILR Press
an imprint of
Cornell University Press
Ithaca and London

First published 2012 by Cornell University Press

Printed in the United States of America

Library of Congress Cataloging-in-Publication Data

The question of competence : reconsidering medical education in the twenty-first century / edited by Brian D. Hodges and Lorelei Lingard.
    p. cm. — (The culture and politics of health care work)
    Includes bibliographical references and index.
    ISBN 978-0-8014-5049-5 (cloth : alk. paper)
    1. Medical education.   2. Competency-based education.   3. Clinical competence.   I. Hodges, Brian David, 1964–   II. Lingard, Lorelei.   III. Series: Culture and politics of health care work.
    R735.Q47   2013
    610.7—dc23   2012013769

Cornell University Press strives to use environmentally responsible suppliers and materials to the fullest extent possible in the publishing of its books. Such materials include vegetable-based, low-VOC inks and acid-free papers that are recycled, totally chlorine-free, or partly composed of nonwood fibers. For further information, visit our website at www.cornellpress.cornell.edu.

Cloth printing   10 9 8 7 6 5 4 3 2 1

For the Wilson Centre: A place that has inspired so
many of us to think and to see in ways not
imagined before we walked through its doors

CONTENTS

FOREWORD

Medical education has been the subject of repeated examinations and in-depth reports about changes that are needed to improve the education of physicians. In 1910, Abraham Flexner wrote a report, funded by the Carnegie Foundation for the Advancement of Teaching, that advocated for changes and promoted standards for medical schools and is credited with changing the way doctors are educated. Perhaps most important, Flexner made medical education a social cause, demonstrating its importance in everyone's life. Flexner's work exposed poor educational content and processes in the preparation of physicians and began what has been a century-long concern with the quality of physician education and practice.

Today, at the beginning of the twenty-first century, the concern with the preparation of physicians continues unabated with significant changes underway in the content, pedagogy, and assessment of physicians and other health care professionals. Two U.S.-based organizations, the American Board of Medical Specialties (ABMS) and the Accreditation Council for

Graduate Medical Education (ACGME), have taken the lead in promoting competency-based training for all physicians.

In addition to the work of the ABMS and the ACGME in the United States, the importance of competence and the attention being paid to it in medical education is reflected in a group of reports that have been published in the past twenty years. Each report defines the qualities and outcomes desired in the "competent" physician. The reports include: *Tomorrow's Doctors* from the General Medical Council in the United Kingdom; the Medical School Objectives Project (MSOP) reports from the Association of American Medical Colleges (AAMC); *Good Medical Practice-USA; The Future of Medical Education in Canada* from the Association of Faculties of Medicine of Canada; *Scientific Foundations for Future Physicians* from the AAMC and the Howard Hughes Medical Institute; and its companion report, *Behavioral and Social Science Foundations for Future Physicians* from the AAMC.

As we see from the focus and titles of these efforts and reports, accountability and responsibility to the public have led to yet another shift in the paradigm of medical education. The key concept in this new paradigm is competence. But just what constitutes competence?

We use many words to define competence—capability, know-how, experience, expertise, aptitude, fitness, skill, and proficiency—but as the title of this book suggests, questions remain about competence. This is why an exploration that provides critical insights into the idea of competence could not be more needed and more timely.

Medical education is now moving from a structured, process-based system that specifies time spent in a classroom or clinical experience (such as a ten-week clerkship in internal medicine) and defines this as the amount of time needed to "learn" the content, to a competency-based system that defines the desired outcome of training, the outcome driving the educational process (such as competence in the ability to take a history and physical examination). The paradigm shift from the structure- and process-based curriculum to a competency-based curriculum and evaluation of outcomes is among the most profound changes in medical education. The outcomes we want from medical education now are physicians who bring a humanistic approach to medicine; who have a patient-centered approach to medical care; an appreciation of the value of fundamental research for the advancement of medical science; a global perspective on contemporary health issues; and an appreciation of the importance of the biological and population sciences for the advancement of medicine. We want practitioners who are able to participate effectively in multidisciplinary and team approaches to patient care; to contribute to eliminating medical errors and improving the quality of health care; and who know how to balance individual and population health needs when making decisions about patient care.

The real challenge for those involved in designing competency-based educational programs is to recognize the complexity of competence as a concept. Only then can they effectively delineate the knowledge, skills, and attitudes that learners must acquire to be able to perform within each domain at a predetermined level and to recognize that the expected level of performance within each domain will vary depending on the learner's stage of education and the specialty he or she is learning. The authors of this book help us do just that. They examine the challenges facing medical education and introduce the concept of "discourse" as a mechanism both for examining the idea of competence and considering how to implement competency-based education. In so doing, they provide us with a new way to ask the questions that are at the heart of every report advocating change, every criticism of medical education, and every conversation that questions why health care is the way it is today.

The chapters in this book range from an exploration of the discourse on cognition and teamwork to the role of emotion in becoming a competent health care professional. The concepts presented in each chapter are rich, even complex, and they are presented articulately and elegantly. Compelling and thought provoking, the essays invite the reader to engage in a range of conversations about competence. The book also provides a comprehensive literature review of the most important work on defining, articulating, and measuring competence. Having all of these references in one place makes for a powerful resource.

This book is rich with new ideas and invites ongoing debate, discussion, and further research (as suggested in several chapters). I hope that the ideas presented in the book will help regulatory organizations and those devoted to assuring the health of the public assess the language and ideas needed to advance the concept of the competent physician/healthcare worker.

Read this book. Share it with colleagues, family, and anyone concerned about the education of future physicians. From the thoughtful reflections of each author, you will learn something new, you will find ideas with which you do not necessarily agree, and you will be thinking about the ideas presented for a long time to come.

M. Brownell Anderson

Acknowledgments

This book would not have been possible without the dedication and thoughtful input of a number of individuals. All of the chapter authors tolerated a punishing schedule of editing with good humor and grace, resulting in the marvelous essays in this volume. The series editors, Sioban Nelson and Suzanne Gordon, skillfully shepherded the book, generously providing advice and guidance throughout. Carla Taines brought careful attention to every aspect of the book's format and was a wonderful collaborator. Alan Bleakley very kindly reviewed the whole manuscript and provided incisive and helpful commentary. Holly Ellinor assisted cheerfully with formatting at multiple stages. Finally, each of us was fortunate to have formal support that made this project possible. Brian Hodges was supported by the University of Toronto Faculty of Medicine, the University Health Network, and the Richard and Elizabeth Currie Chair in Health Professions Education Research at the Wilson Centre for Research in Education. Lorelei Lingard was supported by the Department of Medicine and the Centre for Education Research & Innovation, both at the Schulich School of Medicine and Dentistry, University of Western Ontario.

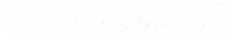

ABBREVIATIONS

AAMC	Association of American Medical Colleges
ABIM	American Board of Internal Medicine
ABMS	American Board of Medical Specialties
ACGME	Accreditation Council for Graduate Medical Education
CBME	competency-based medical education
CEX	clinical evaluation exercise
CIHR	Canadian Institution of Healthcare Research
CME	continuing medical education
CVP	central venous pressure
EI	emotional intelligence
EPR	electronic patient record
ESR	electron spin resonance
IPC	interprofessional collaboration
IPE	interprofessional education
KBE	knowledge-building environment
MOC	maintenance of competence

MSOP	Medical School Objectives Project
OSATS	objective structured assessment of technical skills
OSCE	objective structured clinical examination
PBLI	problem-based learning and improvement
PFL	preparation for future learning
SBP	systems-based practice
SPS	sequestered problem solving
SSHRC	Social Sciences and Humanities Council of Canada

THE QUESTION OF COMPETENCE

Introduction

Brian D. Hodges and Lorelei Lingard

> Every way of seeing is also a way of not seeing.
>
> KENNETH BURKE, *Permanence and Change*

In the past decade, *competence* has grown to the status of a "god term" in medicine and in many other health care disciplines (Burke 1935): an idea with such power that it readily trumps other, competing ideas to shape our educational values and decisions in innumerable—and often invisible— ways. It is, hands down, the governing notion underpinning our sense of what medical education should be striving for in the twenty-first century, overshadowing other popular notions including simulation, objective assessment, professionalism, and patient-centeredness.

The Origins of the Idea of Competence

Almost ten years ago, the shift from a traditional content-based curriculum to a competency-based curriculum was called the "Flexnerian revolution of the 21st century" (Carraccio et al. 2002). This in spite of the fact that competence broadly, and competency-based education specifically, are both old and evolving ideas, much debated in higher-education institutions and in the professions. Calls for competency-based education go back more than half a century (Grant 1979). Competence-based education has been defined as a form of education that derives a curriculum from an analysis of a prospective or actual role in modern society and attempts to certify student progress on the bases of demonstrated performance in some or all of the aspects of that role (Grant 1979). The movement has infused the educational mind-set of a wide range of disciplines, including management (Albanese 1989), psychology (Rubin et al. 2007), engineering (Dainty, Cheng, and Moore 2005), health care (Anema and McCoy 2010; Fullerton et al. 2001; Long 2000), teacher education (Houston 1973), and music (Madsen and Yarbrough 1980).

Predicated on the rise of behavioral objectives in the 1960s and 1970s, the competency-based education movement was originally driven by the need for greater accountability in training, the desire to support students to progress at their own pace, and the call to ensure that training programs were relevant to the goals of society (McAshan 1979). These drivers remain influential today. For instance, the Educating Future Physicians Project of Ontario, which resulted in the CanMEDS competencies for medical education, was driven by a perceived need for medicine to be more accountable to the needs of society (Whitehead, Austin, and Hodges 2011). Because of this, the development of competency frameworks, such as Can-MEDS and the competency model for general practice in the UK, commonly involves a process of seeking public input (Patterson et al. 2000).

Within medical education, the argument for competency-based education has been under way for over fifty years (McGaghie et al. 1978). Recently, however, the wider social-accountability movement has breathed new life into the debate (Leung 2002). As Sullivan (2011) has argued, accreditation bodies now expect professionals to demonstrate that they are indeed achieving what they set out to do. Competencies and outcome-based education are measures that the profession has adopted to better regulate itself in the context of public concerns about patient safety, differential access to care, and the medical profession's struggle with the increasing complexities of practice. What counts as competence is evident in the ways in which programs are structured and in the accountability processes that are implemented around them.

It is hard to find a single health care reform initiative that has not given significant attention to the process of health professional education, which is, in turn, linked to fostering the "competencies" thought necessary for practice in environments that are increasingly complex and stressful in the face of twenty-first-century political, economic, and technical demands. While there are ongoing concerns about "competencies hype," their operationalization in a clinical apprenticeship model of education (ten Cate 2005), and the challenges they present for reliable and valid assessment (Jefferies et al. 2011; Lurie, Mooney, and Lyness 2009), there is no question that the idea of competence has effectively taken over the way we think about medical education goals and enact its curricular strategies. Within universities and other organizations that determine health professional curricula, hardly a discussion or meeting takes place in which competence is not central to the agenda.

The Ubiquity of the Idea of Competence

Competency frameworks now underpin (Simpson et al. 2002) all of medical training in the Western world. These include the Outcome Project of the U.S. Accreditation Council for Graduate Medical Education (ACGME 2011), the General Medical Council's Tomorrow's Doctor (General Medical Council 1993), the Scottish Doctor (Simpson et al. 2002), and the Canadian CanMEDS (Frank 2005) framework. The latter has enjoyed global uptake in countries such as the Netherlands and Australia (American Medical Association 2010a). Similar frameworks are beginning to proliferate globally (Stern, Wojtczak, and Schwarz 2006; Zaini et al. 2011), with implications for global human-health resource strategies and international medical education partnerships.

The idea of competence has proliferated conceptually as well as geographically. There is apparently no limit to the domains in which competence language is relevant. In addition to the usual suspects—clinical competencies such as medical expert and communicator—a range of candidate competencies have been promoted in recent years. In fact, as universities and their affiliated teaching hospitals recognize that attention to patient safety, team-based practice, lifelong learning, and the ability to understand and navigate systems are crucial to the delivery of safe and effective care, "new" competencies have become the lingua franca. Recent entries include science competency (Association of American Medical

Colleges-Howard Hughes Medical Institute Committee 2009), patient-safety competencies (Walton and Elliot 2006), cultural competence (Taylor 2003), and humanitarian response, interestingly advocated as "the competency of competencies" (Hein 2010).

Not only geographically and conceptually pervasive, the idea of competence participates in some of the most critical debates in medical education. It has entered the medical school admissions discussion, offered as an improved candidate-selection strategy (American Medical Association 2010b) to ensure that the "right" individuals get through the gate into the medical profession. It also features prominently in accreditation; for instance, it governs the Liaison Committee on Education's (LCME) standards for accrediting North American medical schools, particularly in relation to standard ED1, which outlines a medical school's responsibilities to define objectives that guide curriculum content and evaluation strategies (LCME 2011). Competence is also arguably the backbone of the past decade's wildly popular global medical education movement, whose agendas not only reflect national concerns but also respond to global forces. Reflecting the rise of a global economy in human resources generally and health human resources specifically, medical schools are embracing a global orientation and marketing their programs to students from around the world. Driven by a need to generate revenue, many medical schools have established contracts to sell services, curricula, or offshore, co-branded campuses to other countries.

Competence is also at the epicenter of the burgeoning field of medical education research and policy development. Competence rhetoric underpins investments in centers for research and development in health professional education around the world. More than twenty peer-reviewed journals publish a swath of literature dedicated to the pursuit of competence in the health professions. When health professional educators and researchers gather together nationally and internationally, competence is always an invited guest at the head table. For example, at the 2011 meeting of the Association of American Medical Colleges (AAMC) in Denver, Colorado, which attracted over four thousand participants, presenters sought to engage the audience by employing titles such as "Competency-Based Medical Education: The Time-Dependent 'Gestational' Approach vs. Milestone-Dependent 'Developmental' Approach," "Do New Models for Early Clinical Experience Produce More Competent Students?" and

"Toward Achieving Competence across the Continuum of Medical Education." A session on "Core Competencies for Collaborative Practice" aimed to "define foundational competencies for interprofessional collaborative practice," tying this imperative to patient-centered care and quality outcomes (AAMC 2011).

Similarly, the nearly three thousand participants from more than seventy different countries who attended the 2011 Association for Medical Education in Europe Conference (AMEE) in Vienna, Austria, could attend more than twenty different sessions with "competence" in the title and many more oriented around the topic (AMEE 2011). The same pattern can be found in programs of the Asia-Pacific Medical Education Conference, held annually for over five hundred medical educators in Singapore, and the International Ottawa conferences, held every two years on a different continent, and attended by more than two thousand health professional educators from around the world. Both feature numerous sessions that focus on competence and its many offspring, including "competency frameworks," "competence-based curricula," "competence assessment," and the like. Not only are academic seminars, keynotes, and workshops devoting large amounts of time to discussing variations on the theme of competence, but entire regulatory, licensure, and certification organizations around the world owe their existence to it.

The Debate about Competency-Based Medical Education

As the revolutionary rhetoric surrounding it suggests, the competence "turn" in medical education promises—and threatens—to change both the work medical educators do and the physicians we graduate. Which is why this book could not appear at a more timely moment. Any idea with the kind of power that "competence" currently wields in medical education deserves careful, critical attention. In the field of health professions education, there are many books and articles on how to *do* competency-based education. Many educators and researchers are also debating the wisdom of competency-based medical education, with some supporting and others challenging it. Supporters emphasize the transformative potential of competency-based education. One critical transformative point regards the tradition of "time-based training," which medical educators have been chafing against in recent years in the face of the problems of physician shortages, physician education debt, and patient wait lists.

Competency-based training is promoted as a solution to this complex problem and, perhaps not surprisingly, surgeons are taking the lead in educational experiments to test this theory. The Royal Australasian College of Surgeons' new Surgical Education and Training program, which commenced training in 2008, is competency based and shorter than any designed previously (Collins et al. 2007). Innovators at the University of Toronto are trialing a competency-based pathway as a solution to the problem of homogeneous postgraduate training regimens that can be prohibitively long and constraining to high performers Their competency-based pathway experiment is promoted as facilitating the fast-tracking of individuals who can show steep learning curves with all aspects of surgical competency (Grantcharov and Reznick 2009).

Critics point to the history of competency-based education in other professional fields and caution against the application of an approach based in technical and vocational fields to the complex, judgment-based profession of medicine. Arguing that the whole is more than the sum of the parts, detractors warn against the atomism, emphasis on routine skills, teaching-to-the-test, and checkbox-driven assessment that are common to competency-based approaches (Huddle and Heudebert 2007; Malone and Supri 2010). Competency-based education has been likened to "tyranny" (Brooks 2009) and to "striving for mediocrity" (Brawer 2009). Educators have worried that it promotes "monkey see, monkey do" education (Talbot 2004), and that it may have "incapacitating effects" on learners (Grant and Murray 1999) and focus our attention on minimum requirements (Bleakley, Browne, and Bligh 2010). Regarding the last point, some argue that preparation in the professions attends almost exclusively to the knowledge and skills required, paying minimal attention to the profession's social ends and civic foundations (Colby and Sullivan 2008). Furthermore, while the drive to turn things into competencies may suit operational and instrumental skills, it is not only insufficient when it comes to more complex and relational aspects of medicine, but may in fact be a dangerous wrong turn motivated by a "lust for assessment" (Wear 2008).

In 2009, an international theory-to-practice consensus conference on competency-based medical education (CBME) was convened by the Royal College of Physicians and Surgeons of Canada (Frank et al. 2010). This group reviewed the broad educational literature to comprehensively lay out both "the promise and the potential perils" of this approach for the future of medical education. They characterized the promise of CBME in terms of its commitment to outcomes, potential for learner-centeredness, de-emphasis of time-based training, and promotion of portability in health human resources. Perils include CBME's threat of reductionism, emphasis on lowest common denominator, tendency toward utilitarianism, and the potential logistical chaos of a progress-at-your-own-pace model. Offering redefinitions of key terms, the group recognized the transformative potential of CBME and called for ongoing debate about its utility and impact.

Another peril not as explicit in this report is the way in which competency definitions, lists, roles, and frameworks may, inadvertently or purposefully, transport purposes and values from their original setting to other settings (in time or in place) where those purposes and values may have invisible or unintended consequences. That is, the language of competence is not only descriptive but also constructive. Eraut (1994, 159) explains that "definitions of competence . . . may be designed for one purpose, and in practice serve quite a different purpose. . . . The definition of what in practice was meant by 'competence' reflected the political purpose it was intended to serve." A 2011 analysis of the origins of the CanMEDS roles framework provides an illustration of the political purposes that may underpin definitions of competence; similarly, the energetic commentary this analysis prompted reveals that much is at stake in both the definitions themselves and the assertion of political purposes underpinning them (Sherbino et al. 2011; Whitehead, Austin, and Hodges 2011).

Debates about "competence" also have arisen in the globalizing world of medical education (Hodges et al. 2009). A case in point is the flurry of activity aimed at developing "global standards" for medical competence (Institute for International Medical Education 2002; Karle 2006). This push to identify a shared, global definition of competence or to operationalize global competence in one set of standards or roles is a logical extension of a global medical education market, but it raises the critical question of who decides what these elements of global competence are. Writing about medical education, Bleakley, Brice, and Bligh (2008) have raised a concern articulated by social scientists more generally (Navarro 1999) that the dominance (economically, culturally, linguistically) of particular countries or regions is almost certain to lead to the marginalization of priorities, values, content knowledge, and exposure to learning contexts of less dominant countries or regions. The dominance of language requires particular attention. If one is to take seriously writing since the mid-twentieth century about the "linguistic turn""—the shift in many scholarly disciplines that foregrounded the constructive function of language—how does one think about "universal standards" expressed in only one language? Ho and colleagues at the University of Taipei have conducted research showing that the construct of "professionalism," a construct operationalized almost entirely in English-language medical education journals, is a subtly but crucially different notion when seen through the language and cultural filters of Taiwan. A greater emphasis on competence as an individual trait in North America as opposed to competence as a collective trait in Asia is just one of the nuances that renders a universal definition of a competence like "professionalism" difficult (Ho et al. 2011).

The Unique Contribution of This Book

While some debate the pros and cons of competence-based medical education and others explain how to achieve various competencies, the authors of the seven chapters in this book offer something very different. Together, the essays in this volume offer something new to the scholarly discussion of competency-based medical education. They do not mount philosophical arguments for or against embracing the idea of competence in medical education. They do not join instrumental debates about how to do competency-based medical education. Instead, they critique the very notion of competence itself and attend to how it has shaped what we pay attention to—and what we ignore—in the education and assessment of medical trainees.

In differing ways, the leading medical education researchers who have contributed to this book all argue that we have only just scratched the surface of developing a sophisticated concept of competence with our various frameworks, taxonomies, checklists, and the like. Indeed, the risk is that as these lists get longer and longer, incorporating ever more diffuse elements, the word "competence" will actually stand in for so many things that it will come to represent nothing at all. While much attention has been paid to the operationalization of competence (and in particular the development of assessment tools), not enough has been paid to the fact that there are some dramatically different paradigms or "discourses" about what competence actually *is*. The goal of this book is to look critically and thoughtfully at several of these different conceptions, or "discourses," of competence and to analyze the educational, moral, political, and scientific implications of adopting certain of these over others. To that end, the seven chapters in this book explore concepts of competence from a range of disciplinary perspectives.

The first chapter, "The Shifting Discourses of Competence," by Brian Hodges, begins with the observation that if one reads the history of medicine, or any of the health professions, it is obvious that the elements used to define competence have changed considerably over time. Competencies move on and off lists of sanctioned and appropriate professional activities for various reasons that include advances in the science, but also include economic, political, and sociological factors. Analyzing the five key discourses that are used to conceptualize medical competence in North America today—knowledge, performance, psychometrics, reflection, and production—Hodges explores each in terms of the implications for learning, assessment, relationships, and the nature of educational institutions. Inspired by a Foucauldian genealogical approach, Hodges dissects the interrelations and power dynamics making each discourse possible. Finally, Hodges reflects on the practical and ethical dilemmas that students and teachers face if they are prepared to accept the notion that competence is a constantly shifting construction.

In chapter 2, "Rethinking Competence in the Context of Teamwork," Lorelei Lingard considers the health professions' traditional approach to competence as something that individual practitioners acquire, perform for assessment, and seek to maintain over their practice life. This individualist discourse of competence does not equip us well to address team situations, particularly those in which individually "competent" health professionals combine to form an "incompetent" team. She reviews the conventional, individualist discourse on competence that underpins much health professional education specifically—and Western culture in general—considering its theoretical origins and the ways in which it inclines medical educators to attend to some things and ignore others. After introducing a more emergent discourse that characterizes competence as a shared and distributed construct, she weighs the implications of viewing competence through both lenses. What kinds of education and assessment might be possible if our conventional discourse of competence were extended? How would such an extension challenge our traditional approaches to "measuring" and "maintaining" competence?

In the third chapter, "Perturbations: The Central Role of Emotional Competence in Medical Training," Nancy McNaughton and Vicki Le-Blanc explore the role of emotion as an integral, and often underappreciated, component of competency in the health professions. The authors bring two different scientific perspectives to the discussion. One perspective views emotion as a social construction, influenced by sociocultural processes. Viewed from this perspective, we would discover a better understanding of the nature of emotion and its relationship to competence through studying social processes, including the way that certain emotions come to be acceptable or unacceptable and, therefore, come to be associated with competence or incompetence. The second perspective views emotion as a neurobiological phenomenon that is related to other cognitive functions such as attention, memory, and decision making. Using this lens to understand how emotion affects competence means measuring cognitive and neurophysiologic variables such as performance, emotion, and salivary cortisol levels. The authors compare and contrast the implications of using each of these different approaches to understanding emotion and its relation to education and practice.

In chapter 4, "Competence as Expertise: Exploring Constructions of Knowledge in Expert Practice," Maria Mylopoulos problematizes a commonly held view—that excellence in the education and training of future *experts* is crucial to the success of all professions—by exploring developments and debates in the conceptualization of *expertise*. She reviews the extensive literature on expertise over the last half century, pointing out that the understanding of expertise has recently expanded to include previously unexplored facets of expert performance. In particular, scholars and researchers are increasingly revisiting the role of knowledge in expert development and practice. Mylopoulos thus analyzes various cognitive constructions of expertise, with a particular focus on the differing ways in which the role of accrued knowledge has been conceptualized in models of expert development and practice. Her chapter discusses key implications of the various treatments of knowledge in theories of expertise for those seeking to understand competence through the lens of expert performance.

In the fifth chapter, "Assessing Competence: Extending the Approaches to Reliability," Lambert Schuwirth and Cees van der Vleuten ask the question, what makes an assessment of competence a good assessment?

Traditionally, assessment of competence has been viewed as a sort of psychological test, by which student characteristics that are not directly visible can be captured through the indirect measure of proxy behaviors. Quality criteria for assessment methods, therefore, are based on those used for psychological tests, the most well-known being reliability and construct validity. Reliability is expressed as reproducibility of the outcomes of the assessment tool—for example, had a group of students been given another test of equal difficulty on the same topic, would they then have obtained similar scores? Validity is understood to be a marker of whether the test actually measures the characteristic it purports to. Both criteria are currently determined using psychometric formulas applied to numerical data. Yet there are major limitations to the assumption that all elements of competence must be inferred from the numerical scores on reliable and valid tests. The authors argue that many current competence assessment instruments do not fit well into this paradigm. They contend that, to properly assess competence, subjective human judgment and qualitative language-based data are required. With the understanding that important decisions made about students must be fair and defensible, they consider the challenge associated with finding subjective assessments that meet high quality standards. These challenges notwithstanding, however, the authors address the urgency of exploring new directions in the assessment of competence.

In chapter 6, "Blinded by 'Insight': Self-Assessment and Its Role in Performance Improvement," Kevin Eva, Glenn Regehr, and Larry Gruppen examine the foundations on which many modern theories of self-improvement are built. From athletic coaches to business leaders, there is a general belief that the path to better performance involves "looking in the mirror" to openly and honestly identify one's weaknesses and take steps to improve on them. With the health professions as perhaps the most extreme example, the industry's current models of maintenance of competence and self-regulation seem to be formalizations of the instruction "Physician, know thyself." The authors caution against reliance on self-assessment of competence.

While each of us has more information with which to judge our own abilities than is available to external observers, Eva, Regehr, and Gruppen argue that it is this very wealth of information that may prevent us from generating accurate impressions of our own abilities. The authors review research that raises questions about the adequacy of self-assessment, explores reasons why inadequate self-assessment may actually be adaptive, and looks at the many ways in which we can all fool ourselves into believing that we have privileged insight into our own capacities. Their chapter raises fundamental concerns about the way in which the health professions typically conceive of self-assessment and the purposes for which it can be productively and reliably applied. The chapter concludes with a description of the way in which models of professional self-regulation can be effectively modified, given the evidence base that has accumulated to date.

In the seventh chapter, "The Competent Mind: Beyond Cognition," Annie Leung, Ronald Epstein, and Carol-Anne Moulton examine competence as the "moment-by-moment" activities of health care professionals. Popular opinion would have us believe that experts, through appropriate and exhaustive training, "just have the answer"; they simply "know what to do" and "know how to do it." The authors in this chapter, however, question this reassuring assumption. While it may be true for many daily activities, they argue that professionals are unable to stay in this "automatic" mode all the time. By virtue of the complexities of professional practice, there will necessarily be times of uncertainty—when the usual rules might not apply or when knowledge does not seem adequate.

During these moments of practice, experts must transition out of the routine mode and into the more effortful mode of thinking: in fact, they engage in "slowing down when they should." Leung, Epstein, and Moulton argue that these slowing-down moments mark the more critical moments of professional practice. From this, they ask: How can experts monitor their activities to ensure they make the transition when appropriate? What are the influences on them as professionals during these moments, both cognitive and social, that may prevent them from slowing down appropriately? Bringing together literatures on reflection and mindfulness that inform the phenomenon of slowing down, the authors examine the initiators and influences of this transition and explore ways that expert physicians "stay out of trouble." Calling into question the concept of automaticity in expert professional activities, they explore the role of mindful practice as an alternative way of remaining attentive.

Mindfulness is precisely what this book brings to the issue of competence. As so many have pointed out, the idea of competence is indeed one of the biggest shifts in medical education since the Flexner Report. Because of the power of this idea, it is critical that we understand the notions and assumptions underpinning it; that we highlight the dangers of unthinking acceptance of the idea of competence and all its attendant frameworks and taxonomies; and that we critically consider its impact on prelicensure education, professional practice, and continuing professional development and recredentialing. In the history of medicine, some very popular ideas have turned out to be gods with feet of clay, which is why this latest "god term," competence, deserves close and careful scrutiny. We invite readers to join in this scrutiny, to be challenged by the ideas in this book, and to contribute to a critical debate about what we see and don't see in our current ways of looking at, and for, competence in medicine.

1

THE SHIFTING DISCOURSES
OF COMPETENCE

Brian D. Hodges

Competence Is a Shifting Construct

Competence is a word that is so frequently used, in so many different ways,
that it risks having no meaning at all. As mentioned in the introduction,
Lingard (2009, 625) has called *competence* a "god term," a word so weighty
that its mere use trumps other considerations. To articulate the need for
better tools for the assessment of competence is to invite a concerted nod-
ding of heads. But what *is* competence? A common approach to this
question is to concretize the term in a list of skills and attributes that presumably, taken together, define competence. A more recent and increasingly popular approach is to define a set of roles that professionals should
play and to think of competence as the degree to which individuals fulfill
them. Some think of competence as a capacity. Others imagine competence
as an attitude to deepening one's expertise. More provocatively, some argue
that competence is neither role, trait, capacity, nor attitude but a mechanism tied up in the way professional groups maintain their status in society.

No matter how it is understood, there is no escaping the centrality of discourses of competence to health professional education and practice. Rather than being distressed by the diverse definitions and disparate uses of the notion of competence, in this chapter I turn the lens around and explore how various definitions—emphasized at different times and in different places—can help us better understand the nature of health professional education itself; that is, I explore the way in which competence is defined as a means of shedding light on the way in which health professionals conceptualize our role in society, our relationship to other professions, and our *professionalization project*. Here, then, I wish to look at competence, not in its unity, but in its dispersion.

If we read a history of medicine, or of any health profession, it is rapidly apparent that the practices accepted as competent change considerably over time. Indeed, it seems we live in an era marked by particular urgency to pin down the specific competencies that belong to and define each of the health professions. This can lead to some interesting and occasionally amusing conflicts. Reeves, Fox, and Hodges (2009) recount a skirmish between nurses and nutritionists over which profession *owns* the competence of breast-feeding, dividing up the woman's breast into the process of breast-feeding latch (nurses) and the nutritional value of breast milk (nutritionists). Amusing anecdotes aside, historical study reveals that competencies have moved on and off lists of activities sanctioned by each profession with regularity, partly as a result of advances in the science but also for economic, political, and sociological reasons (Hodges 2005; Shorter 1985).

An oft-cited example is the competence of delivering babies. Today, medical students assume that delivering babies has always been a core competence of physicians. This is not the case. In the early nineteenth century a *competent* physician gave purgatives and performed bloodletting, but certainly did not deliver babies. That was a core competence of midwives (Shorter 1985). Yet in only a few decades, physicians in Scotland managed to shift the competence from midwifery to medicine, arguing that physicians were the only professionals competent to independently deliver babies. A similar history played out in the United States where between 1900 and 1930 physicians added obstetrical practices, traditionally provided by midwives, to their list of competencies. Gieryn, Bevins, and Zehr (1985) explain that this shift resulted from a combination of tactics that included physicians depicting midwives as unscientific and therefore risky while simultaneously lobbying for government licensing programs to reduce the range of services that midwives could legally provide. Witz (1992), recounting the same history, adds that the key means physicians used to adopt the competence of delivering babies from midwives was to incorporate delivery onto a list of physician competencies and then assess it on medical licensure examinations.

While it may seem common sense to argue that something appears on a medical licensure examination because it is an established domain of medical competence, this example illustrates that sometimes things can become competencies *because* they are codified on a list and then tested on examinations. Similar historical examples can be found in anesthesia (once the province of nursing) and prescription medications (once the province of pharmacists). Witz (1992) emphasizes that this phenomenon is not specific to the medical profession, nor is it simply about doctors appropriating skills from other professions. Rather she sees the space between professions as a sort of semipermeable membrane, subject to forces that allow competencies to move back and forth from one group to the other. This uptake and download of competencies (in her analysis the structure is vertical because of the dominance of some professions over others) is in constant ebb and flow at the professional boundaries. Particularly active *boundary work* can be observed, for example, between nurses and nursing assistants; physical therapists and massage therapists; radiologists and radiology technicians; physicians and physician assistants. In medicine, boundary work has characterized the relationship of family physicians and specialists ever since the two divisions of medical practice emerged.

This constant redefinition of the content, skills, attitudes, and aptitudes that characterize competence is the purpose and focus of this chapter. However, I am interested less in *which* elements should or should not be part of professional competence than in *how* specific activities or domains come to be associated with competence and to belong to particular professions in different times and places. The significance of such an analysis is not simply to amuse historians and sociologists of the professions. The definition and operationalization of competence is a very high-stakes activity. Competence frameworks act as barriers to entry (by predefining traits and attributes necessary for study); affect progression (forming the basis of in-training evaluation); and are implicated in graduation, certification, and licensure (determining the content of examinations) and processes of discipline and maintenance of certification. Each of these mechanisms is becoming more and more codified and rigorous in the United States, Canada, the United Kingdom, and other countries around the world. I am also particularly interested in the ethical dimensions of creating powerful high-stakes admissions, assessment, certification, and licensure examinations for domains that are subject to such frequent shifts.

Competence Is Constructed by Discourses

Viewed from a traditional scientific background, my approach may appear strange. What does it mean that medical competence is "constructed" by discourse? The concept is perhaps more readily understood when looked at from a long historical perspective. An exercise I find useful is to examine archival images of physicians over several centuries. I was first inspired to think about how dramatically the image of competence has changed when I came across the *Book on the Physician Himself* (Cathell 1890). Published at the end of the nineteenth century, the book is filled with advice for newly graduated physicians on how to appear competent. Much emphasis is placed on proper appearance (a three-piece suit and a walking stick with a silver head), office decoration (a reflection of one's *station in life*), and behavior in society (such as never being seen alone with young women or *undesirables*). Of course, at that time in history, few effective medical treatments were available and the European practices of physical and laboratory examinations were just being adopted in North America (Shorter 1985). The author seemed not to be embarrassed about advising graduates that their *image* of competence would be created more through gentlemanly dress and particular social habits than any aspect of actual practice. Deep in the library stacks, I found a dusty book with images of a physician galloping through the night on horseback. Presumably the doctor was racing to enact some heroic measure, such as removing an appendix on a patient's kitchen table, a fatal intervention that terminated the short life of my own great-uncle at the turn of the last century. Perhaps the doctor's skill in horseback riding exceeded his facility with a scalpel, but his sweaty gallop through the night nevertheless conveyed something about competence, at a time when there were no operating rooms or anesthetics to be had in the countryside. On the Internet, meanwhile, I found old images from the television show *Marcus Welby, M.D.* that ran during the 1960s and 1970s. No longer wearing a three-piece suit and certainly not on horseback, this character dressed in a white coat. His confident demeanor conveyed an air of competence, reinforced by the starched creases of his lab coat—a piece of clothing reserved at that time for doctors alone. Physicians of Marcus Welby's time, of course, considered it appropriate, professional, and presumably competent not to tell dying patients that they were dying (for fear of worrying them), to call up the male head of the household to talk about the health of his wife or children (of any age), and quite possibly to appear in advertisements to promote a brand of cigarettes.

While these seem like caricatures today, they are helpful to illustrate how behaviors and attitudes associated with competence have changed rather dramatically. These changes occurred because the construction of medical practice and of medical competence also changed. Of course a good bit of this evolution is the story of science. Certainly, the doctor who sniffed a patient's urine as a diagnostic test in the nineteenth century did not have the benefit of laboratory analysis. Operating on the kitchen table in the early twentieth century was necessary because of the absence of adequate operating theaters and modern anesthesia. We may even be prepared to excuse the 1950s physicians who promoted cigarette smoking as being simply unaware of the yet-to-emerge science underlying the dangers therein. These changes do indeed correspond to the advancement of science. But what of strolling around the wards in gentlemanly attire and expecting the nurses to stand at attention? How about talking to a woman's husband instead of the patient herself about her illness? Is there a link to the end of these practices (which surely would now seem bizarre, unprofessional, and incompetent) and the fact that women, who were once thought to be too feebleminded to pursue studies in science (Strong-Boag 1981), now represent more than half of most medical school classes? What about withholding the truth from a dying patient? Today, changing values rather than scientific advances mean that respecting a patient's autonomy is linked to competent, professional practice. Finally, is it science that has made it unlikely that we would see a doctor promoting smoking, or is it more related to questions about the ability to practice competently while using addictive substances or while beholden to a contract to advertise products for industry?

These dimensions of professional competence reflect a set of cultural expectations and norms that are constantly shifting. Historical perspective is helpful to "make strange" things that we take for granted today (Kuper and Hodges 2010). Another way of examining socially constructed practices is to look at our context from the vantage point of another culture. Think of this as reverse anthropology. Many years ago I attended the wonderful presentation of a researcher from south Asia who "went to a land called Florida to live among the cheerleaders" for a year. Taking photos and making anthropological observations about a practice as familiar as cheerleading turned it into something exotic and interesting for riveted audiences in India, but also in the United States.

In a similar vein, imagine holding a debate with doctors from different countries of the world as to whether talking to a woman's husband about her health is "competent" behavior or not, and what regional, national, cultural, or other variations would be reflected in the answer. Or more simply, ask your colleagues or friends why it is important for a doctor to wear a white coat rather than a three-piece suit or jeans. The question "What is appropriate dress for a doctor?" always leads to spirited debates depending on one's generation, specialty, or geographic location. During my years as an examiner with a U.S. specialty board I recall attending a required "cultural sensitivity training" session. We were warned to be careful about holding stereotypes about competence that could be associated with the way people dress in different parts of the United States. A candidate from Hawaii wearing a floral-patterned short-sleeve shirt and sandals, for example, might appear less competent to an examiner from New York, where the uniform of competence (at least for an exam) is a blue suit. Southerners, on the other hand, might well be chewing gum and have long red fingernails and a big beehive hairdo, according to the presenter. I was glad of this latter bit of advice when my second candidate appeared just that way.

Stepping back from our own culture can help us see the constructed nature of things we assume to be *natural* or *normal*. Certain North American practices seem unusual, even bizarre, to those from other places. For example, a colleague visiting my university hospital from the Philippines commented recently that she found it sad that the patients in our intensive care unit had *no family*. She was shocked to learn that rather than valuing the constant presence of family members at the bedside, we instead regulate their presence with something called visiting hours. In many countries, the family is present at the bedside twenty-four hours a day and during all discussions with the health care team. This is one of several examples I have written about that illustrates how practices that become normalized among health professionals can seem bizarre to anyone encountering the hospital and its culture for the first time (Hodges 2010). Consider that we make people take off their clothes, walk around in public spaces wearing a half-open blue gown, refer to them loudly in the third person with labels like "the fracture in room 5," and introduce ourselves as "Hi, I'm Ortho." These practices strike the uninitiated as part of an unusual, and not particularly respectful, culture.

Foucauldian Discourse Analysis Is Helpful to Understand Shifts in Competence

The notion that competence is not a fixed entity may be unsettling to those accustomed to the positivist research tradition. Positivism is characterized by assumptions of fixed, objective phenomena that can be confirmed through empirical study. What positivist approaches leave unexplored, however, are the political, cultural, and economic contingencies in particular times and places that make it possible to think in certain ways, say certain things, and act, dress, carry oneself—in short, to *be*—a particular way.

Rather than framing all developments as part of a continuous line of progress, researchers taking a critical, constructivist view emphasize power, equity, and justice, forces that can hardly be said to follow a continuous and linear upward slope (Kincheloe and McLaren 2000). In the words of Starr (1982, 3–4), "The dream of reason did not take power into consideration.... The history of medicine has been written as an epic of progress, but it is also a tale of social and economic conflict over the emergence of new hierarchies of power and authority, new markets and new conditions of belief and experience." Seen through a critical constructivist lens, not all changes in society, and therefore in health care or professional education, are progressive or even rational. Good and bad ideas and practices come and go (Calhoun 1995), shaped by the political, social, and economic imperatives of the time. These imperatives can be unearthed by studying what Michel Foucault called *statements of truth:* strongly articulated arguments about what is true/untrue, just/unjust, legitimate/illegitimate, permitted/forbidden in a given place or time. Statements of truth are the surface manifestation of deeper and more complex systems of *discourse*. Discourse used in this Foucauldian sense is a highly useful way of thinking about the ebbs and flows of competence. I think of the *discourses of competence* as all of the current linguistic (speech and text), behavioral (performance and appearance), and material (architectural, institutional) representations of what it is to be a competent professional at a particular time in history or in a particular place. *Discourse analysis* thus involves paying attention to how these elements systematically construct particular versions of the social world (Rogers et al. 2005).

I previously conducted a discourse analysis about competence examinations. This involved semistructured interviews in the United States, Canada, and the United Kingdom and the analysis of hundreds of published articles (Hodges 2009). Since then I have had the opportunity to reflect on the specificity of these Anglo-Saxon discourses and compare them with discourses used in other countries of the world such as China, Denmark, Ethiopia, Israel, Japan, Jordan, New Zealand, Pakistan, and Poland. More formally I undertook, with French colleagues, a preliminary comparison study of the discourses of competence in Canada and France (Segouin and Hodges 2005). These analyses involved characterizing some of the major discourses in use in medical education, today and in the past, by paying particular attention to recurring key words, metaphors, and conceptions. I was then able to delineate the roles created for students and teachers as a result of the dominance of certain discourses. Finally, I was able to describe how different discourses have led to increases or decreases of power for various organizations and institutions.

During the analysis of examination discourses, I collected information related to discourses of competence more generally. Ultimately, I identified discourses related to competence (*knowledge, performance, psychometrics, reflection,* and *production*). Below I present a detailed description of each of the five discourses.[1]

For each I have selected a representative symbol and an associated name. Though I do not mean to imply that these named individuals alone created the various discourses, their names and ideas do appear frequently

---

1. An earlier, simplified version of these descriptions of the discourses of knowledge, performance, psychometrics, and reflection appeared in the paper "Medical Education and the Maintenance of Incompetence" (Hodges 2006).

TABLE 1. Symbols, Roles of Teachers and Students, and Common Measures of Competence Associated with Five Discourses

Discourse of competence	Symbol	Role of teacher	Role of student	Common measures of competence
Knowledge discourse	Harrison's textbook	Providing facts and knowledge; elaborating mechanisms	Reading and memorizing facts for recall	Knowledge tests; often multiple-choice questions
Performance discourse	Miller's pyramid	Teaching skills; creating simulations; making observations	Practicing and demonstrating skills	Performance-based assessments; observed "real" or simulated scenarios
Psychometric discourse	Cronbach's alpha	Shaping student characteristics and behaviors toward a "norm"	Adapting self to required "norm" so as to maximize data points on standardized measures	Standardized scales and rating; often checklists
Reflection discourse	Schön's reflective practitioner	Guiding introspection; mentoring; acting as "confessor"	Reflecting and demonstrating self-assessment and self-regulation	Portfolios; reflective exercises
Production discourse	Taylor's scientific management	Managing the production of a quality product	Conforming to the standards of quality	Quality control measures; audits

in association with each discourse. The symbols also provide a form of shorthand to facilitate the discussion of the discourses and their interrelations. The five discourses and their associated names and symbols are as follows (see table 1):

1. Knowledge discourse: Harrison's textbook (Kasper 2005) and competence-as-knowledge
2. Performance discourse: Miller's pyramid (Miller 1990) and competence-as-performance
3. Psychometric discourse: Cronbach's alpha (Cronbach 1951) and competence-as-reliable-test-score
4. Reflection discourse: Schön's reflective practitioner (Schön 1987) and competence-as-reflection
5. Production discourse: Taylor's scientific management (Taylor 1911) and competence-as-product

Knowledge Discourse

> [A]ll but the very brightest students are submerged by the torrent of
> information. It is no wonder if they say "I have so much to remember,
> I have no time to learn."
> (Dornhorst 1981, 513)

Knowledge discourse is characterized by use of the words facts, foundational knowledge, basic science, first principles, fund of knowledge, classic textbooks, classic articles, and multiple-choice tests (see table 2). In this discourse, the role of teacher is to be a source of wisdom, and teachers' main activities revolve around helping students receive or elaborate knowledge. Core teaching activities are didactic lectures and seminars that aim to transmit knowledge. The most common measure of competence-as-knowledge is a written test, often consisting of multiple-choice questions. This combination of teaching and assessment methods requires students to memorize and reproduce information, and much time is spent reading. The ideas, roles, and activities associated with the notion of competence-as-knowledge construct a competent individual as one who can memorize, reproduce, and elaborate on large amounts of factual data. This age-old conception is based on the idea that the accumulation of knowledge is linked to, and indeed central to, competence. For thousands of years, in

TABLE 2. Key Words, Concepts, and Theoretical Foundations Associated with Five Discourses

Discourse	Key words	Concepts	Theoretical foundations
Knowledge discourse	Facts, foundational knowledge, basic science, first principles, fund of knowledge, classic textbooks, classic articles, multiple-choice tests	Competence is based on the mastery of a body of complex and specialized knowledge.	Contemporary: cognitive science; ancient: monastic scholarship
Performance discourse	Simulations, simulated patients, feedback, performance, skills, OSCE, multiple observations	Competence is revealed through observable behaviors and the performance of skills.	Contemporary: behaviorism; ancient: dramatic arts
Psychometric discourse	Reliability, validity, generalizability, data, psychometricians, candidates, checklist, item banking, cut point, standardization	Competence is captured via the conversion of human attributes and behavior to numbers using reliable and valid psychometric measures.	Contemporary: psychometrics; ancient: mathematics
Reflection Discourse	Reflection, self-directed learning, learning contracts, portfolios, adult learner	Competence is manifested and ensured through self- reflection, self-assessment, self-regulation	Contemporary: self-actualization, psychoanalysis; ancient: philosophical/religious introspection/confession
Production discourse	Cost, production, finished product, accountability, outcomes, efficiency	Competence is a product resulting from processes that are productive and efficient.	Contemporary: production/capitalism; ancient: alchemy

cultures as diverse as classical Greek, Roman, Arabic, and Chinese societies, the memorization and mastery of vast amounts of information was required for scholars in diverse fields. In Western cultures, this knowledge discourse has roots in the monastic traditions of memorizing and reproducing religious books.

After the 1960s, however, in the United States, George Miller (1990) and other medical educators began to argue that too much emphasis on knowledge risked creating knowledge-smart doctors who had poor interpersonal and technical skills. Jacques Barzun argued in the *New York Times* that a preoccupation with doing well on recall tests "conditioned the way young people in America think" (1988, 27) and that they have "better-developed cognitive abilities to recognize random facts than to construct patterns or think systematically" (ibid.). Critics continue to argue that an overemphasis on knowledge discourse may lead to incompetence as a result of the poor integration of knowledge in practice, a lack of appropriate interpersonal behaviors, and poor technical abilities.

Performance Discourse

> In many places they would ask students to write an essay on the origin of the word shoelace, or give them a multiple choice question on the design of shoelaces or even ask them to describe the steps in tying a shoelace. Whereas really the only way of doing it is showing you know how to tie a shoelace.
>
> (R. Harden, cited in Hodges 2009, 76)

Performance is observed. In psychological terminology, performance relates to *behavioral* aspects of human activity. Performance thus has less to do with cognitive processes and more with action, movement, speech, and gesture, though behaviors are also often used as proxy indicators of underlying attributes (personality) or abilities (cognitive reasoning). In the behaviorist tradition, performance can be learned or modified through practice, repetition, and the iterative loop of performance-feedback-performance. Integral to performance discourse is an observer or observers who may simply watch, or who may critique or evaluate. Given the strong tie to practice, performance discourse often invokes methods of simulation because it is cumbersome or unreasonable to perform the same behaviors repeatedly in clinical settings. The goal of those who use performance discourse is the shaping of behaviors in desired directions and a significant emphasis is placed on *formative* teaching and assessment methods. Performance has a long history in the dramatic arts. Epistemologically, performance discourse is linked to early-twentieth-century schools of behaviorism (Skinner 1953) and sociological concepts of the presentation of the self (Goffman 1959). The emergence of behaviorism in medical education was associated with shifts of power in medical schools in the late twentieth century when curricular reforms led to significant reductions in the teaching of basic sciences. As clerkships were lengthened, the teaching of *how-to* aspects of medicine, such as interviewing and physical examination, gained in both curricular time and importance. As clinician-educators acquired more control of curricula, it was a natural extension of their own focus on *doing* in clinical practice to shift teaching and assessment in medical schools toward performance and away from memorization of facts and mechanisms.

Performance discourse is associated with a very different set of words from that of knowledge (see table 2), including simulated patients, feedback, performance, interaction, patient-encounter, communication and interpersonal skills, and observation. In this discourse, the role of the teacher is to demonstrate and observe skills. Competence is measured with performance-based assessments that require students to demonstrate what they can do. This discourse has been associated with the development of a wide variety of new testing methods including paper and computer-based problems, simulated patients, objective structured clinical examinations (OSCEs), and their many variants. Such a combination of teaching and assessment methods creates a role for students to perform for observers, with much time spent practicing (Hodges 2003). Miller's (1990) pyramid contains a conceptual taxonomy that places knowledge at the bottom of a pyramid and a sequence of performance verbs—"knows, knows how, shows how and does" (S63)—at increasingly higher levels on the pyramid. These ideas, roles, and activities construct the competent individual as one who is able to demonstrate communication, interpersonal, physical examination, and other skills for observers in structured, often simulated environments.

Although performance discourse remains prominent today, beginning in the 1990s cognitive psychologists and sociologists, approaching the issue from different perspectives, began to articulate worries about too much emphasis on competence-as-performance. Leading the cognitive perspective, Norman (2005a) argued that "cracks started to appear in the pyramid," citing research evidence that "knowledge wasn't quite so low down and skills quite so high up as one might have thought" (85). Schuwirth and van der Vleuten (2006) and Eva (2003) argued that content-specific knowledge is essential for real-life problem solving and that both knowledge and problem solving are highly domain specific. The strong interdependence of skills and knowledge, so-called *content specificity* of knowledge, means that teaching content-free, generalizable, performance skills is problematic. Sociologists, meanwhile, have argued that an overreliance on simulation training, often employed in response to decreased availability of real patients, might encourage students to become *simulation doctors* who act out a good relationship with their patients but have no authentic connection with them (Hanna and Fins 2006). Thus, argue these two groups of critics, an overemphasis on performance discourse may actually lead to incompetence, characterized by poorly integrated knowledge on one hand and fake performances on the other.

Psychometric Discourse

> In proportion as it becomes definite and exact, this knowledge of educational products and educational purposes must become quantitative, take the form of measurement. Education is one form of human engineering and will profit by measurement of human nature and achievement as mechanical and electrical engineering have profited by using the foot-pound, calorie, volt and ampere.
>
> (THORNDIKE 1922, 1)

Psychometric discourse began to have prominence in medical education in the United States during the 1980s and is very much present today. Linked to psychology on one hand, and statistics, measurement, and evaluation on the other, psychometric discourse was created and advanced in tandem with the evolution of two new roles for individuals to play: the arrival in medical education of *educational psychometricians* and the transformation of simulated patients into *standardized patients*. Psychometrics aims to represent human characteristics and behaviors with numbers for comparison purposes. Central to this approach is the use of statistical methods to identify a *true score* (the presumed numerical equivalent of a real phenomenon) and the control or elimination of *variance,* sometimes referred to as *statistical noise.* In the 1980s, a series of shifts—including a drive for accountability, the growth of large testing institutions, and an influx of medical educators with training in measurement and evaluation—led to the rise of this new discourse that focused on psychometrically reliable tests as a central means of defining competence. *Cronbach's alpha* (Cronbach 1951) became a widely used statistical measure of the reliability of test scores.

Psychometric discourse is characterized by words such as reliability, validity, generalizability, data, psychometrician, candidate, checklist, item banking, cut point, and standardization (see table 2). More recently, accountability imperatives and legal ramifications in the United States and Canada mean that in some places more attention is given to high-stakes tests at the end of training than is allotted to in-training assessment and formative feedback.

The need for multiple sampling and standardization means the role of teachers is driven toward presenting repeated and relatively homogeneous examples of clinical materials and cases so that students can eventually maximize their scores on tests. Reducing variance fosters a drive to normalize the elements (be they knowledge, skills, or attitudes) measured. In some countries, private organizations have sprung up to offer training that paying students hope will improve their chances for high scores for admission or on medical school examinations. In particular, employing binary or multipoint checklists and ratings in a wide range of tasks such as performance assessments (OSCEs, oral examinations), in-training assessments, and the assessment of values, attitudes, and professionalism means removing items that do not contribute to the overall reliability of a test. In an interesting discursive nuance, the word *discrimination* is used in a positive sense in psychometric discourse. Thus, test questions or rating-scale items that "do not discriminate between test takers" are removed. Reducing the *variance* of performance-based assessments by standardizing the examiners, performances, appearance, and demographic characteristics of patients, and calibrating raters to use measurement tools in the same ways, may contribute to the loss of authenticity of teaching or examination problems, cases, and scenarios.

For students, the psychometric discourse acts as a driver to activities that they perceive will maximize their eventual in-training and examination scores, reduce their variance, and approximate what they perceive to be the desired *norm*. Taken together, this set of ideas, roles, and activities constructs a competent individual as one who can adapt him- or herself in such a way as to achieve high scores on standardized measurement instruments by thinking, speaking, or behaving in ways that conform to the expected norm.

While this discourse is currently very prominent, critiques are emerging (Kuper et al. 2007). Schuwirth and van der Vleuten (2006) have written, "We dismiss variance between observers as error because we start from the assumption that the universe is homogenous, where in fact the more logical conclusion would have been that the universe is more variant" (298). In addition to the loss of authenticity associated with standardization, one of the side effects of stringent adherence to standardized norms is an apparent discriminatory effect on experts. Those who are skilled in creative problem solving or pattern recognition, or who simultaneously gather information and manage problems, or who use other nonstandard approaches (nonstandard in the sense that they are not likely to be reflected in the step-by-step algorithms) may achieve low scores on standardized, detail-oriented checklists. For example, a study conducted at the University of Toronto showed that clinicians with the most experience actually scored lower on previously validated OSCE checklists than residents or medical students did (Hodges et al. 1999). Further, concerns about the security of high-stakes testing has meant that where psychometric discourse is dominant, feedback to students may be very limited.

Thus an overemphasis on psychometric discourse may result in incompetence as a result of encouraging overly normalized and standardized characteristics and behaviors and discouraging the use of pattern recognition, integration, and synthesis. Increasing standardization in processes such as admissions risks a reduction of student diversity and, during the in-training years, may lead to the suppression of marginal and potentially creative, innovative characteristics, behaviors, and approaches. Essentially, what is not counted or measured does not exist.

Reflection Discourse

The concept of learner as a mere processor of information has been replaced by the image of a self-motivated, self-directed problem solver.
(Ministry of Education, Ministry of Colleges and Universities 1980, 2)

In the mid-1990s, Donald Schön's book *The Reflective Practitioner* (Schön 1987) became popular in medical education circles. Perhaps this occurred in part because the introspective, self-focused nature of reflection functioned as something of an antidote to the hard, objectified regimens of external, standardized testing. The reflection discourse is characterized by words such as self-directed learning, insight, learning contracts, portfolios, and adult learners (see table 2). In this discourse, teachers take on roles as guides or mentors, or what might be called *confessors*. A common measure of assessment is portfolios, and the use of reflective exercises such as diaries, reflective essays, and learning contracts is popular. Many professional certification and licensure organizations require practicing clinicians to submit a self-directed learning portfolio as evidence of maintenance of competence. Taken together, this set of ideas, roles, and measures constructs a competent individual as one who engages in a trinity of self-reflection, self-assessment, and self-regulation (Hodges 2004). These concepts have roots in the mid-twentieth-century popular psychology notion of *self-actualization,* which itself originated in psychoanalysis. Further back, notions of introspection and confession derive from philosophy and religion. Why such ideas should have emerged with force in medical education in the late twentieth century is not entirely clear. It may be, as Ronald Epstein (1999) has argued, that the profession was rediscovering the central role of *mindfulness* in competent medical practice. Despite the apparent individualist, self-directed quality associated with reflection and introspection, however, the adoption of reflective techniques in relation to maintenance of competence may represent a more subtle and distributed form of professional regulation.

As with other discourses, there are emerging critiques of reflection discourse. One thrust can be summarized by the words of Jeremy Taylor, the seventeenth-century cleric who is said to have commented: "It is impossible to make people understand their ignorance, for it requires knowledge to perceive it; and therefore, he that can perceive it, hath it not" (Pickett 1857, 1). In more recent research Davis et al. (2006) confirmed this worry in their analysis of seventeen studies comparing doctors' self-assessments against objective, external reviews. They reported that in most studies there was a subset of clinicians who were unable to judge their knowledge or skills accurately (Davis et al. 2006). This work is consistent with the studies of Kruger and Dunning (1999) showing that, in a whole host of areas of competence (problem solving, logical reasoning, humor), a significant proportion of individuals demonstrate a wide gap between assessments of others and assessments of themselves. This gap persists even when opportunities are given to observe performances of other individuals and to reassess their own. These findings were replicated in a study I undertook with colleagues in which family medicine residents were asked to manage a case of child abuse. Among those who scored very low on management, knowledge, and interpersonal skills, there were several who rated themselves substantially higher than the observers. When they were given an opportunity to watch a variety of others handle the same situation and then rescore their own performances, the inflation of self-ratings persisted (Hodges, Regehr, and Martin 2001). Regehr and Eva (2006) have gone further, arguing that the notion of self-assessment itself may not be valid. Such findings raise questions about reflection discourse and competence.

From a sociological perspective, there have also been critiques of reflection discourse. Nelson and Purkis (2004) argue in relation to nursing that "reflective practice provides the mechanism whereby nurses internalize the new professional ethos of self-government" (250), but that "regulators appear quite unconcerned about the lack of coherence between what is being monitored 'at a distance' and the actual professional knowledge [needed] to function skillfully and competently" (256). Thus an overemphasis on reflection discourse runs the risk of rewarding individuals who *appear* to be reflective, but who may have deficiencies in knowledge, skills, or attitudes that are not directly measured.

Production Discourse

> The training of physicians in America has changed from that of a mentor/ apprenticeship relationship to one in which students are part of an impersonal, mass production process.
>
> (Farnsworth 1991, 1005)

Production discourse rose to prominence in medical education in the 1990s. It is very much a dominant discourse today. Production discourse is imbued with language and concepts borrowed from manufacturing and industry. Key words that characterize this discourse include cost, production, finished product, accountability, outcomes, and efficiency (see table 2). In this discourse, the role of the teacher is as part of a larger productive institution, the goal of which is to convert raw materials (students) into a quality finished product. The notion of assessment shifts slightly to the idea of *quality assurance*.

The origins of production discourse can be found in Frederick Taylor's (1911) *Principles of Scientific Management*. Taylorism was widely taken up in industry and manufacturing at the dawn of the twentieth century. Taylorism introduced standardization to the work environment and to the tasks of work and of the workers themselves, with an overall goal of increasing efficiency in the service of productivity. Taylorism became a significant part of many kinds of organizations at the beginning of the twentieth century, and it has been continuously refined and reinforced by corporations for the last seventy-five years (Becker and Steele 1995). The uptake of these principles changed the organizational aspects of the workplace: "The corporate order, with its assembly-line techniques, job differentiation, and increased organizational size, demanded a different type of office space and a more regulated and regimented flow of time" (Kwolek-Folland 1994, 107). Many of the twentieth-century changes to the workplace and to the nature of work itself can be traced back to Taylor and scientific management. Production discourse is at the heart of capitalism, but it might be suggested that there are more ancient metaphorical roots. The idea of creating value from raw materials through controlled means was also the goal of alchemists.

As we have seen, the psychometric discourse had already begun to emphasize a need for standardization, though for reasons of better statistical analysis. In production discourse, standardization has even greater prominence; education is construed as a manufacturing process and students as raw material first, and then product. Several objections are raised about an excessive use of production discourse in medical education. These include the overemphasis on outcomes and surveillance that can distort student learning; the creation of high-stakes assessment of "quality" that produces no feedback to advance learning; and the commoditization of teaching and testing that leads to significant shifting of costs to students. Thus an overemphasis on concepts of productivity and the metaphors of education as manufacturing can lead to new forms of incompetence resulting from the dehumanizing of education and paradoxically a reduction in "quality" of education environments in a drive for efficiency and lower "per unit" cost.

The Emergence and Interrelationship of Discourses

To this point, I have presented the five discourses as though they were discrete entities: circumscribed ways of thinking, speaking, and behaving.

For teaching purposes, I sometimes liken the five to islands that one could visit on a sea voyage, much like an anthropologist visits and observes new and strange lands. But of course this is a fiction. All five discourses are in active use in medical schools today and each of us moves between them. My interest, therefore, is not to argue for the relative merits of one or another discourse (I don't *believe* in reflection discourse more than I *believe* in performance discourse, for example) but rather to stimulate critical thought as to why certain discourses, and their attendant adverse effects, come to be dominant at certain times and in certain places. It may be interesting to ask, "Is *knowledge* of neurotransmission more important than *performance* of a neurological examination?" or, "Is *reflecting* on losing one's temper with a patient more important than *scoring* in the ninety-fifth percentile on a communications objective structured clinical examination with an interstation reliability of 0.8?" But these are not the questions that interest me. Rather, I am interested in how the discourse of knowledge came to dominate over half of the medical curriculum following the Flexner reforms (Flexner 1910); why performance eclipsed knowledge in the latter part of the twentieth century; for what reason self-analysis and reflection permeated all levels of teaching at the end of the twentieth century; and why it is possible to say that only an examination with psychometric reliability is appropriate to certify competence.

Perhaps rigorously designed empirical studies will one day tell us with certainty whether lectures or problem-based learning are more effective; whether test-enhanced learning or portfolio-based reflection make a better doctor; whether adhering to strict quality assurance standards at graduation is better than accepting people with particular attributes into medical schools; and whether any of these factors lead to noticeably different or better health care. But I suspect that no amount of experimental, controlled, and positivist research will provide satisfying answers to many of these questions. I think it is more interesting to ask why these questions are posed in the first place, seeking to understand the emergence and uptake of different paradigms of education as well as the positive and negative effects of each.[2]

---

2. An earlier analysis of the interrelation of the discourses of performance, psychometrics, and production appeared in *The Objective Structured Clinical Examination: A Socio-History* (Hodges 2009) and is reproduced here in an expanded form, incorporating the discourses of knowledge and reflection.

Discourses are not naturally occurring entities; they are created by people and institutions and are wrapped up in power, hierarchy, and struggles for legitimacy, funding, jobs, and turf. To study their rise and fall it is necessary to understand the source of their discursive legitimacy. Put more bluntly, if it can be said that "the competent physician is _____," the research questions are: Who says so? On what basis do they justify this statement? And what power authorizes them to say this is true? In this way a sort of family tree, or *genealogy,* can be created for each discourse by studying its emergence and staying power. For example, we can find out when the first performance-based assessment took place, when medical educators first started to write about reflection, or when the first psychometric criteria for competence were used. Then the points of dominance and the ebbs and flows of the explanatory power of each discourse can be characterized. Finally, the relationships between discourses can be examined.

It is important to underscore that the discourses I have presented here are not unique to medicine. While a sort of *origin* can be determined for each discourse, at least inasmuch as it is possible to locate moments when each first appeared in the literature or in the speech and writing of medical educators, I do not want to imply that these moments of emergence were unique to the education of physicians or even health care. While the discourse of performance in medical education rose to prominence in the 1960s, for example, performance discourse was not invented in medical education. Rather, it is a discourse that was imported from behaviorism, an epistemology dating to the early twentieth century and the work of B. F. Skinner (1953) and others. Psychometrics emerged in medical education in the 1980s but was a well-established discourse in psychology in the United States as early as World War I (Hanson 1993; Rose 1985). Reflection and introspection have long histories in both Western and Eastern philosophy and punctuated the development of psychoanalytic thinking in the late nineteenth century. Medical educators did not tap into this discourse in a substantial way until well into the last decades of the twentieth century. Finally, while production discourse is strongly emerging in medical education at the present time, it is being imported from a much broader arena of economic activity associated with neoliberal global capitalism born during the Industrial Revolution.

There are also interesting interrelationships between the discourses. Knowledge discourse—the idea of mastery of vast swaths of information—is probably as old as scholarship itself. Performance discourse, on the other hand, was not adopted in medical education until the 1960s when universities throughout North America and Europe were rocked by student demonstrations and calls to tackle hierarchy and oppression. New ways of thinking about the purpose of educational institutions, teachers, and students, and about how and why knowledge is constructed led medical schools to reexamine and reinvent the nature of teaching, assessment, and the role of patients in medical education. Some of the inventive efforts to change the medical classroom (such as the use of prostitutes and actors to teach, for example) represented dramatic departures from traditional medical teaching (Godkins et al. 1974).

The use of performance discourse rapidly shifted, however, from the classroom to testing and examinations. As I have detailed elsewhere (Hodges 2009), Howard Barrows, for example, was initially unable to interest medical leaders in the use of simulated patients for teaching in California in the 1960s, though he attracted somewhat greater interest when he moved to McMaster University in Canada in the 1970s. When he modified his performance discourse slightly to argue that simulations could be used to produce better *examinations* of competence (adding psychometric discourse to his performance discourse), his ideas were taken up (Wallace 1997). It seems to me that the roots of performance discourse are less to be found in the 1960s movement to address power differentials in the classroom and more in another force that rose to prominence in the 1960s: the imperative to render new domains of human activity *scientific*. So-called *soft* aspects of medical practice (the doctor-patient relationship, empathy, communication skills) were given the same attention as the *harder* elements (scientific knowledge) through efforts to measure and quantify them. The creation of simulation technologies was a further logical development to bring what were previously loosely controlled dimensions of physician performance under scrutiny.

Psychometric discourse did not replace performance discourse so much as it transformed it. It is interesting to ponder why psychometrics was not taken up in any meaningful way in medical schools when it first emerged in North American universities after World War II. Of course part of the answer, as we have seen, is that the influx of psychometricians into medical schools did not occur until the 1970s (Kuper, Albert, and Hodges 2010). It is possible that these developments were connected with the end-of-century transfer of power and funding from public institutions to the private sector (Teeple 2000), requiring greater accountability and measurement that subsequently led to the rise of national testing bodies (Dowdle 2006). In the United States and Canada in the 1980s and 1990s, health services and educational institutions were privatized and tuitions deregulated, while measures of university and hospital outcomes became priorities. We may wonder, however, why psychometric measurement earned a much less prominent place in certain countries of Europe, where some medical educators are now calling for new psychometric models (Schuwirth and van der Vleuten 2006).

Psychometric discourse then paved the way for the emergence of production discourse. Psychometricians originally aimed for standardization and reduction of statistical variance to increase the reliability of the analysis of performance. But it was a small leap to the standardization of everything related to teaching and testing, including the roles of employees, the design of institutions, and the behavior of teachers and students. This small leap was medical education's adoption of principles of manufacturing. By the late 1990s, the movement of goods and services within, but also between, countries meant that the reduction of costs and the efficiency of production became priorities (Teeple 2000). As medical school classes increased in size around the world, pressures for efficiency made the discourse of business and manufacturing attractive. Most recently, medical education production discourse has taken on global dimensions with attempts to develop international standards for accreditation and assessment (Hodges et al. 2009). The universalization of Anglo-American models of medical education, such as the establishment of U.S. medical schools and examination models in countries where production costs are lower, is a new development associated with globalization (Segouin, Hodges, and Brechat 2005).

On the surface, reflection discourse appears to be a reaction to the rigid standardization of psychometrics, the excessive external testing associated with knowledge and performance discourses, and the dehumanizing effects of conveyor-belt production. For some, introspection and reflection conjure up images of individual freedom idealized in midcentury North American writing about *self-actualization*. Foucault and others have noted, however, that *technologies of the self* may represent subtle but powerful means of governmental power. I have argued previously that *guided* self-reflection and the confessional aspects of reflection may be aspects of new models of professional control (Hodges 2004). Nelson and Purkis (2004) argue that the shift to competence-as-reflection for the purpose of maintenance of certification may also represent a new form of governmentality linked to the need for professions to guard their turf from an ever-encroaching threat of public regulation on one hand, and the boundary skirmishes with sibling health professions on the other.

Of What Value Is a Discourse Perspective on Competence?

> As every medical professor knows, you just find a patient with some fractures and escort a gaggle of students to the bedside for a good long stare. As long as the sufferer is not prodded too hard, or denied a clear view of the television, no ethical rules are violated.
>
> (*Economist* 2007, 77)

The discourses that medical schools use to understand and shape medical competence come to bear directly on the approaches chosen for teaching and assessment. Medical educators increasingly recognize that the curriculum, both formal and hidden, has a lifelong impact on students (Hafferty 1998). *The Economist* used the above quotation to draw attention to the fact that the roles played by students and teachers are not always ethical. Poking and prodding an objectified patient, sometimes without his or her consent, reflects a particular construction of roles and distribution of power and authority for patients, doctors, and their students in our society. All five of the discourses we have examined create a way of thinking and being for students in relationship to their future role as a doctor. They also create ways of thinking and being in relationship to their teachers, their patients, and the institutions in which they work. It is here that the ethical implications of the use and interplay of various discourses are most profoundly felt.

Just as painters balance inherent tensions between surface and depth, detail and perspective, illumination and shadow, medical educators must blend together different proportions of knowledge, performance, testing, reflection, and production from the discursive palette. Very different curricular canvases result. An overemphasis on particular dimensions can result in the emergence of unexpected views of incompetence, inharmonious interpersonal hues, or jarring ethical patterns.

While doctors are very thoughtful about the ethical implications of medical practices and treatments of patients, and are particularly concerned to warn patients and families about side effects of procedures and medications, the same cannot be said for educational interventions. Yet, as I discussed above, teaching and assessment methods also can have important side effects. Because teaching and assessment methods are selected on the basis of a particular discourse about what competence is, it follows that we can trace a relationship between different discourses of competence and unwanted side effects produced by specific teaching and assessment methods linked to them.

Table 3 summarizes together some of these adverse effects. The forms of *recognized* incompetence shown arise directly from the constructions of competence that flow from each discourse. For example, in knowledge discourse, competence is constructed and measured as the memorization and recall of factual information. Incompetence, then, is the inability to memorize or recall factual information. As I have shown, however, this pairing of competence/incompetence (ability/inability to memorize facts) renders invisible other forms of competence/incompetence (ability/inability to communicate, ability/inability to reflect, etc.). Additionally, table 3 describes the nature of teacher-student, and student-patient relationships that will be emphasized when each discourse is emphasized.

The implication of this line of reasoning is that attention should be given to the hidden forms of incompetence associated with dominant discourses. For example, where reflection discourse and portfolios are prominent, monitoring for a gap between reflections and actual skills should be a priority. Or where performance discourse makes simulation training prominent, it may be wise to remain vigilant for the appearance of pseudoempathy. In this way, medical educators can be more attentive to the emergence of unhelpful or incompetent cognitive, behavioral, or attitudinal dimensions similar to the way in which physicians monitor for adverse drug reactions. An additional conceptual shift is necessary, however, to adopt such an approach. Medical educators would have to consider that problematic cognitive, behavioral, or attitudinal phenomena may be less the responsibility ("fault") of individual students than the creations of the medical school and the health care institutional environment and its exigencies. This notion is consistent with Hafferty's (1998) description of the *hidden curriculum*.

TABLE 3. Constructions of Competence, Adverse Effects, and Relationships Associated with Each Discourse

Discourse	How incompetence is defined in this discourse	Adverse effects that might result from overemphasis of this discourse (hidden incompetence)	The nature of relationships associated with this discourse
Knowledge discourse	Inability to recall facts and information	Stronger ability to recognize random facts rather than to interpret patterns or synthesize contextual information. Poor interpersonal or technical skills.	Strictly, learning knowledge alone does not require a patient or a teacher. The teacher's role, when in contact with students, is transmission and elaboration of information. Learning relationships may be solitary, dyadic, or large group.
Performance discourse	Inability to perform	Lack of integration of relevant knowledge with performance. Inauthentic skills, such as superficial displays of pseudoempathy or cursory examination skills.	By nature, performance requires an observer. Here a patient (real or standardized) is central and an observer/teacher is present. Learning relationships are triadic.
Psychometric discourse	Inability to score highly on checklists/standardized measures	Prolongation of novice behaviors (shotgun data collection) and lack of development of expert reasoning and behaviors. Inability to address the vagaries and variance of real contexts. Homogenization/suppression of diversity. Impoverishment of teacher-student relationship and the loss of feedback.	Data gathering is central and collection is dispersed (multiple sampling). Thus observing/scoring raters and standardized patients are diffusely present and may be anonymous or at a distance. Learning relationships are diffused and one-way surveillance is common.
Reflection discourse	Inability to produce convincing self-assessment	Superficial self-assessment that masks inability to detect or address deficiencies. Development of reflective abilities alone in the absence of knowledge and skills.	Like knowledge discourse, in its pure form reflection does not require a patient. The intent is to reflect on patient interactions, but the material attended to is virtual/reflective. Learning may be solitary with periodically dyadic relationships.
Production discourse	Inability to meet the standards of quality assurance/audit	Commodification, dehumanization of teaching and testing technology. Power shift from teachers/classroom to testing organizations, sometimes to corporations.	Relationships (with patients or teachers) are not central. A more anonymous surveillance monitors student activity and output. Learning relationships are dispersed and subsumed by one-way surveillance.

Conclusion

> There are times in life when the question of knowing if one can think
> differently than one thinks, and perceive differently than one sees, is
> absolutely necessary if one is to go on looking and reflecting at all.
>
> (FOUCAULT 1990, 8)

I have argued that discourses are not simply spontaneously created entities that emerge like shooting stars from a dark night. Discourses emerge because there are important sociological, political, economic, and cultural contingencies that make them possible, indeed necessary. Discourses are associated with power. The dominance of one discourse over another has significant implications for what is considered legitimate, what positions are made available for individuals, what will get published, what will be funded, and which institutions will gain power and influence.

Take, for example, the combative discussions about the role of basic sciences in medical education. Though there is little debate that medicine has something to do with knowledge of anatomy, physiology, and histology, the question of how much of these subjects is necessary causes some problems. Things get a bit fuzzier when we talk about biochemistry and organic chemistry, and while advocates of Latin and materia medica have long disappeared from the scene, anthropology and sociology are pushing from the margins. A question much debated is, which domains of knowledge and skill are most important to the practice of medicine? The struggles that play out at curriculum committee meetings often have more to do with which departments and which faculty members dominate medical schools than the competencies needed for practice. While dominant discourses of competence have something to do with the training and practice of future generations of doctors, they also have a lot to do with curriculum time, funding, prestige, and legitimacy of whole swaths of the professoriat.

Approaching competence as a sociohistorical construction with links to power can free us from simply reproducing old arguments, stale turf battles, and recurrent boundary skirmishes: in short, various *discourses* constrain our thinking. By rejecting the idea that physician competence is linked to the naturally unfolding development of a profession that is advancing in tandem with scientific discovery, it is possible to see that ways in which appropriate professional behaviors are defined may also be linked to economic and political reasons in the play of power (Foucault 1977).

My goal for this analysis is not simply to nudge the reader into a paranoid state by convincing you that all acts of curriculum reform and examination are games of power played out on a field of domination. Rather, after Foucault, I argue that discourses and power are *productive* (Gordon 1980). That is, understanding the ebbs and flows of power and harnessing them can have very positive effects. I believe that there are two major advantages to having exposure to the sort of multipolar, discursive analysis that I have presented here. First, the ability to move between different discourses at the macro level is much like using the biopsychosocial model that so many of us value at the patient level: it encourages multidimensional thinking. This flexibility of approach is good for students and it is good for teachers. I suspect it is also a core attribute of successful administrators and leaders. Second, the project of creating a new admissions policy, implementing a new course, or reforming a whole curriculum will surely founder on the rocks of resistance if change leaders are not well versed in the political, social, historical, and economic dimensions of their undertaking.

Finally, accepting competence as a shifting construction, buffeted by the forces of dominant discourses, has implications for faculty development. Bleakley, Bligh, and Browne (2011) contrast the faculty development required to support early-twentieth-century structural and scientific reforms of medical education with what is required in the twenty-first century to reorient medical education socioculturally. The latter change, they argue, requires development of a corps of medical educators and clinical teachers who have a strong grasp of the importance of identify formation, the play of power, and the centrality of context, in additional to pedagogical skill. I agree with these authors that medical educators of the future need more than manuals describing methods of teaching and assessment. What they require in addition are sources that deepen and transform their thinking about the very purpose of medical education. It follows, then, that faculty development in the twenty-first century should give considerable attention to the ebb and flow of the discourses of *knowledge, performance, psychometrics, reflection,* and *production* in medical education.

Rethinking Competence in the Context of Teamwork

Lorelei Lingard

Rarely can a patient's health care needs be met by a single care provider. Patients who go to their family doctor with persistent headaches interact with the physician and the nurse in the office, and may get referred to a specialist or sent to have a diagnostic imaging test. Patients with chronic conditions like diabetes will interact with a number of providers in addition to their family doctor, such as endocrinologists, ophthalmologists, and dietitians. Patients who go to an emergency department with chest pain will be seen by a nurse and an emergency physician, and may also be assessed by a general internist or a cardiologist. And if patients are sick enough to get admitted to hospital these days, they almost certainly have a complex array of clinical needs that require the expertise of a host of specialists, technicians, and allied care providers. Today, more than ever before in the history of medicine, the provision of care is a team sport.

In the public and in the health professions themselves, there is growing recognition that teamwork is necessary for the delivery of high-quality health care (Romanow 2002). Research shows that good teamwork improves the safety of the care patients receive—fewer errors are made, particularly when team members communicate effectively with one another and have a shared plan for what's going to unfold (Gawande et al. 2003; Joint Commission on Accreditation of Healthcare Organizations 2005; Pronovost et al. 2003). Initiatives like the Safer Surgery checklist, which bring operating room team members together both before a procedure to communicate critical details and after to review and improve teamwork, offer proven benefits to patient care, such as improved morbidity and mortality rates (Haynes et al. 2009).

As we've come to understand how important teamwork is to care delivery, governing organizations around the world have developed frameworks to ensure that teamwork is being learned by health professional trainees (Accreditation Council for Graduate Medical Education [ACGME] 2003b; Frank 2005). How is teamwork learned? Currently, it is mostly through socialization: student physicians and nurses learn how to be team members through their experiences on health care teams during their training (Haber and Lingard 2001; Montgomery Hunter 1991). As trainees *try out* being a team member and watch other team members interact, they learn about professional values, professional turf, and collaborative strategies for working with others (Spafford, Schryer, and Lingard 2008). Of course, what trainees learn in this apprenticeship environment ranges from the good to the bad and the ugly: depending on whose behaviors they decide to imitate, new team members could be acquiring attitudes and habits that are not conducive to teamwork. Recognizing that this existing tradition of ad hoc learning is insufficient, policymakers are supporting an interprofessional education (IPE) movement as a key to ensuring that team members learn how to work together effectively (Health Canada 2010). University bodies are declaring a commitment to integrating IPE into their health professional curricula (Association of Faculties of Medicine of Canada 2010; Oandasan et al. 2004), and accreditation bodies are beginning to demand its inclusion in training and assessment strategies for accredited programs.

Clearly, the health professional community has embraced the notion of expert teams as critical to its clinical and educational mandates. We know that good teams deliver better care. And we've identified teamwork as a necessary component of curriculum. Now we face a pressing educational question: How do we approach *competence* in relation to teams?

The Problem

The ideas in this chapter emerge from my study of health care teams over more than a decade. In particular, I have been struck by the incongruity between the way we talk about competence as *something an individual has (or doesn't have)* and some regularly observed phenomena in team research:

1. Competent individuals can come together to form an incompetent team.
2. Individuals who perform competently in one team may not in another team.
3. One incompetent member functionally impairs some teams, but not others.

Our traditional approach to competence as an individual phenomenon does not equip us to grapple productively with these realities of team practice. And the rise of teamwork, as both a core mechanism for quality care and a core mandate for education, means that we cannot afford to disregard the complex intersection between the competence of the individual and the competence of the collective.

Competence is one of health professional education's most cherished ideas. As mentioned in the introduction of this volume, it's what the twentieth-century rhetorician Kenneth Burke would call a "god term" (Burke 1952): a sort of education idol, an "expression to which all other expressions are ranked as subordinate" (Weaver 1953). This god term presides over many of our conversations in health professions education, conversations including curriculum reform, evaluation systems, program accreditation, and maintenance of certification. And, like other god terms of our era (*patient safety* has recently emerged as one, *objective assessment* has long been another), *competence* is a rhetorical trump card, regularly played as the last word in debates about how health professions education should function.

Across the globe, physician competencies have become an increasing focus of medical education at all levels in the past two decades. At the undergraduate level, the Medical School Objectives Project (MSOP) by the Association of American Medical Colleges (AAMC) (MSOP 1999) encouraged educators to think about generic medical student abilities that would translate across medical schools. As early as 1993, the Royal College of Physicians and Surgeons of Canada began the CanMEDS Project, completed in 2005, to identify societal health care needs and define the competencies essential to specialist physicians in Canada (Frank 2005). In the United States, competence vaulted into the foreground of educational policy and practice when the Accreditation Council for Graduate Medical Education (ACGME) and the American Board of Medical Specialties (ABMS) jointly agreed on six competencies for the certification and maintenance of certification of physicians (ABMS 1999; Horowitz, Miller, and Miles 2004).

Using this framework, the ACGME began holding residency programs accountable for implementing competency-based approaches (ACGME 2003b). With this accountability, assessment of the ACGME competencies has become a pressing issue for residency program directors, who must demonstrate that their programs are teaching these competencies and that their trainees are attaining them. While it is becoming increasingly evident that to quantify competencies such as *professionalism* and *communication* in a reliable and valid way is a persistent challenge (Lurie, Mooney, and Lyness 2009), the *idea* of general competencies continues to accrue support as a means for organizing and rationalizing our educational priorities (Ginsburg et al. 2010; Lurie, Mooney, and Lyness 2009).

From a rhetorical perspective, the powerful language of "competence" demands close attention because it both reflects and reproduces dominant values in health professional culture. According to Kenneth Burke, "every way of seeing is also a way of not seeing" (Burke 1935, 70). He drew attention to how words function as "terministic screens": "even if any given terminology is a *reflection* of reality, by its very nature as a terminology it must be a *selection* of reality, and to this extent it must function also as a *deflection* of reality" (Burke 1966, 45 [emphasis in original]). What aspects of competence are we attending to, and what aspects are we avoiding? What actions and values are made possible by our way of seeing competence in health professions education, and what actions and values are rendered impossible? With its central premise that language not only describes but also constructs reality (Burke 1968; Lingard and Haber 1999) rhetoric allows us to trace in the language of competence both our attitudes toward the phenomenon and the actions that emerge as sanctioned by those attitudes.

In this chapter I explore what we mean by *competence* in health professional education, with three goals. First, I draw critical attention to what the god term invokes and what it elides in its conventional usage in our health professions education discourse. Second, I introduce an emergent way of seeing competence that directs educators' attention in different directions. Finally, I consider the implications of adopting both ways of seeing as a means of productively reorienting our education and research agendas.

Our Conventional Way of Seeing

The individualist discourse of competence has pervaded our culture throughout the lifespan of health professional education. Medical education is predicated on individual learning theories such as adult learning and reflective practice, which presume an autonomous learner. It is also strongly informed by cognitive psychology constructs such as memory, problem solving, and decision making, which take as their starting point the individual learner or expert (Regehr and Norman 1996). In fact, the entire medical education enterprise is currently predicated on the individual. We select candidates based on individual academic qualification. We assign individual grades to students, even in the context of group activities such as problem-based learning. We evaluate residents based on objective structured clinical examination (OSCE) performances as individual diagnosticians. We license trainees based on examination of individual knowledge and skill. We monitor licensed practitioners' ongoing development through accrual of individual continuing medical education (CME) credits, and we remediate problematic performance by targeting the individual performer.

This tradition of individualism is not unique to medical education. It permeates Western medicine as a whole and, beyond that, Western culture and philosophy. Gordon has asserted that "naturalism" and "individualism" are the two major traditions shaping Western medicine's dominant values (Gordon 1988). The political and humanist philosophy of individualism asserts "the primacy of the individual and individual freedom" (21); in fact, the individual, Gordon explains, is the central symbol in Western cosmology, enjoying distinct "priority in the individual/society equation" (35). Taking as its starting point the "pure will and reason" of the individual being, individualism "has little use for society and culture" (42). Probe almost any aspect of Western culture and you'll find this pattern repeated: for instance, we define life success in terms of individual progress and gains; our concerns and theories of child development are focused on the individual child; our traditional religious culture is oriented toward individual accountability and salvation.

It is not surprising, then, that individualism pervades the academic and organizational cultures of one of our dominant institutions—medicine. In academic medicine, the promotional structure assigns value to individual achievements, even in a climate of growing collaborative efforts in teaching and research. Similarly, notwithstanding a recent movement toward increased interdisciplinarity by national research funding bodies (Canadian Institutes of Health Care Research 2006), funding mechanisms persist in privileging the individual who holds principal investigator status and many agencies restrict this role to a single researcher (Social Sciences and Humanities Council of Canada 2009). And then there is the clinical billing structure, which is predicated on the actions of individual practitioners, as is the profession's medical-legal accountability structure, even with acknowledgment of collaborative care practices (Canadian Medical Protective Association 2008).

There have been some discussions of the limitations of such an individualist culture for the evolution of medicine in the face of current challenges. One example comes from the domain of safety science, which is concerned with making the practices of medicine's complex care delivery system more reliable and less prone to error. Amalberti, a scientist whose research considers how to make complex systems such as transportation and nuclear engineering safer, has argued that the goal of an "ultra safe" health care system is fundamentally constrained not by economics or science but by cultural values and system barriers (Amalberti et al. 2005). Of the five barriers that Amalberti and his colleagues review, three of them—the need to limit the discretion of workers, the need to reduce worker autonomy, and the need to make the transition from a craftsmanship mind-set to that of equivalent actors—are related to medicine's culture of individualism. These barriers allow individual physicians to determine the degree of risk in their practice, to emphasize their own goals to the exclusion of others', and to embrace idiosyncratic variety rather than standardization of processes. Amalberti's take-home message is that medicine cannot achieve competence as a system until it is prepared to relinquish its prioritization of the individual.

Premises Underpinning the Individualist Discourse

According to Hodges, medical education has defined competence in various ways over the last century: as knowledge, as performance, as reliable test score, and as reflection (Hodges 2006). Each definition has been predicated on the notion that competence is *a quality that individuals possess*. This notion is so commonplace, so deeply ingrained in medical education, that it seems unnecessary, almost silly, to state it. In this section of the chapter I trace the theoretical origins of this idea, the thinking that has made it so matter-of-fact, so *normal* for educators to be concerned about competence as individual knowledge, individual performance, individual test score, and individual (self)-reflection.

This section focuses on three key premises underpinning the individualist discourse of competence in medical education:

1. Competence is a quality that individuals acquire and possess.
2. Competence is context-free, untied to time and space.
3. Competence is a state to be achieved.

Premise 1: Competence Is a Quality That Individuals Acquire and Possess   A fundamental assumption in the individualist approach to competence is that learners come to *possess* knowledge, skills, and attitudes through engagement in various educational activities. It is this notion of individual possession of competence that underpins conventional assessment approaches. From the multiple-choice exam, to the long oral exam, to the OSCE, the purpose of the examination is to see what knowledge, skills, and attitudes the learner possesses, and to have these performed so that objective witnesses can judge the extent and quality of these possessions. Even in assessment settings that reproduce interactive dynamics, such as a telephone interaction between a medical resident and a pharmacist, the group setting is only a provocation for the performance of individual communicator competence.

This assumption of individual possession of competence grows out of the learning theories on which medical education has been based since the late twentieth century. As Bleakley has argued, varieties of adult learning theory, experiential learning, and reflective practice—all popular in recent decades—view the learner as "an active agent resonating with medicine's tradition of autonomy" (Bleakley 2006, 151). In an orientation that privileges the individual actor, knowledge is treated as commodity and private property, and learning is an individual enterprise. "'Autonomy', 'self-directed learning' and 'self-assessment' are then legitimate currency in such an economy…[and are] taken to be self-evidently 'good' and therefore 'true'" (152). Such pervasive individualism influences how medical educators view the key questions, problems, and solutions in their field.

The notion of individual competence fits with medicine's icon of the heroic student, cramming her head full of an astounding amount of knowledge. Interestingly, though, the notion also appears where we might not be expecting it. For instance, it figures prominently in the recently emerged discourse of IPE, a surprising instance, because IPE is not predicated on individual learning theories to the same degree as traditional medical education approaches. IPE, defined as students from diverse disciplines learning *from, with,* and *about* one another, has strong roots in social learning theory, with its emphasis on learning through participation in a community (Oandasan and Reeves 2005). Consequently, to find the notion of individual competence running through groundbreaking conceptual, educational, and policy texts on interprofessional collaboration (IPC) and education (IPE) is something of a curiosity. These texts reflect an individualist orientation in their articulation of a tension between individual professional expertise and collaborative expertise. In fact, there is a core assumption, even in current rhetoric about the importance of teamwork and IPE, that "individual professional expertise is foremost and must be assured" (Sinclair et al. 2007). Current IPE texts are careful to reassure that they are not arguing with or threatening the core value of profession-specific knowledge/skills as an educational priority. Further, there is also a tacit logic that, not only do we need both, but individual expertise needs to necessarily precede team expertise—that you can't learn to collaborate until you possess some core, individual knowledge. Tracing this problem, Bleakley (2006) argues that, even in educational settings where the need for teamwork learning is recognized, the tacit reference is often individual rather than distributed knowing or learning: teamwork is posited as merely a combination of competent individual workers who *possess* appropriate knowledge.

The notion of competence as individually possessed is woven into the mandates and vision statements of almost all the major medical education and assessment organizations in the United States, Canada, and the United Kingdom. Individualism is a logical emphasis in a system where licensure, billing, and medico-legal accountability function on an individual practitioner basis. The tacit logic of individualism pushes us further, however, deflecting our attention from other relevant foci. For instance, the General Medical Council's mandate is "to protect patients from harm—if necessary, by removing the doctor [who fails to meet the public's standards] from the register" (General Medical Council 2010). This mandate expresses the notion that incompetence (and the consequent threat of patient harm) resides *in* a physician, and can be corrected by taking the physician out of the practice system, revealing a key characteristic of the individualist approach—its disregard of context and of the interaction between individual factors such as knowledge, skills, attitudes, and contextual factors such as relationships, temporal/spatial pressures, and multiple conflicting goals. This notion introduces the next premise, which is that competence, as an individual characteristic, acquisition, or possession, is context-free.

Premise 2: Competence Is Context-Free, Untied to Time and Space   The premise that competence is context-free is strongly evident in the recent uptake of competency frameworks used to guide teaching and assessment. In essence, the assumption is that a competent practitioner is *generically* competent—that is, their performance of competence in one situation should predict future performances in other, similar situations. This individualist premise can be traced well beyond medical education's landscape. In a critical review of competencies and workplace learning with particular reference to U.S. literatures, Garavan and McGuire (2001) describe competency as fundamentally an attribute-based concept, an "atomistic, mechanistic and bureaucratic notion" with a strong bias to consider competence as context-free. They argue that this tradition of competence, based in Taylorism and the push to maximal efficiency in production, emphasizes "identifying, measuring and developing behaviors, which will distinguish individuals who continuously outperform others" (146). In business, such an articulation of competence fosters globalization of the workforce, through recognized standards and measures of assessment. In medical education, too, such an approach to competence makes possible the consideration of a global standard, a mobile health workforce, an industry to accredit this workforce, and a climate of international trade and competition in health human resources (Hodges et al. 2009).

Two prominent examples of the influence of this premise can be found in the language of the dominant medical competency frameworks in the United States and Canada: the ACGME core competencies and the CanMEDS roles. In the ACGME Outcomes Project, the *systems-based practice* competency, which is "manifested by actions that demonstrate an awareness of and responsiveness to the larger context and system of health care and the ability to effectively call on system resources to provide care that is of optimal value," seems the most likely to be linked intimately to context (ACGME 2003a). However, this sense of context is a generic, universalized concept of the system. And the behaviors associated with systems-based competency are individual: among them, residents "work effectively in various healthcare delivery settings," they "coordinate patient care with the health care system," and they "work in inter-professional teams." Essentially, the competency is housed in an individual, conceptualized as the effective navigating of their work environment to meet their individual care delivery goals.

The CanMEDS framework includes a *collaborator* role, akin to the ACGME's *system-based practice* competency, but it is conceptualized at the level of the individual, with competencies and enabling competencies characterized as behaviors that individual physicians are able to enact. Within the collaborator competency, "the specialist is able to effectively consult with other physicians and healthcare professionals...and contribute effectively to other interdisciplinary team activities" (Frank 2005, 15). To demonstrate such competency, residents need to show their ability to "participate in an interdisciplinary team meeting, demonstrating the ability to accept, consider and respect the opinions of other team members, while contributing specialty-specific expertise him/herself" (ibid., 9). In the reality of end-of-rotation evaluation, which is often characterized by limited observation of resident performance by faculty (Watling et al. 2008), a resident's demonstration of this collaborator competence in one interdisciplinary meeting (which may be all that an evaluator has available for consideration when s/he completes the evaluation) is taken as being representative of generic competence, and the collaborator skills thus presumed to be good for all such situations. Where multiple observations of performance occur, any differences across multiple situations will be interpreted, at best, as psychometric noise or error in the measurement of the individual's generalizable skill.

The emphasis on individual subject positions and abilities in competency frameworks like the ACGME core competencies and the CanMEDS roles is salient because it positions us to assess individuals for these skills rather than to assess social acts of collaboration. These competencies are assessed through global rating forms that evaluate to what degree an individual resident inhabits and performs the subject position of, for instance, "collaborator." Because the evaluation is of an individual, not of an event, each of these items necessarily reduces the observed social exchange to individual qualities and actions, such as "interacts easily with nurses." The problem is that this approach belies the dynamism and dialogic nature of such an interaction: from one exchange to another, the ease of interaction may vary significantly depending on the relationship between the resident and nurse, their awareness of one another's current state of mind and workload, and how the topic of the exchange intersects with their respective scopes of practice. The nature of the collaboration, therefore, emerges from the contextual features and the relational aspects of the social exchange; however, our existing competency frameworks inevitably boil this down to visible abilities or characteristics of the resident being evaluated. It is not that such boiling down is *wrong;* rather, that it is unavoidable in the context of an individualist approach to competence. And it deflects our attention from relational issues, such as power dynamics, as well as from sources of incompetence, such as an inability to adapt collaborative strategies to new or changing situations.

Premise 3: Competence Is a State to Be Achieved   As Hodges expresses it, "We think of medical education as a process that moves novices from a state of incompetence, to one of competence" (Hodges 2006). By degrees, learners can progress developmentally through stages toward full achievement of this state. Individual learners are vessels that arrive empty of the core knowledge, skills, and attitudes required to practice medicine; medical education is oriented toward providing these ingredients and measuring how much of them each vessel contains as it progresses through the levels of training. Following years of classroom and apprenticeship learning, learner-vessels exit the educational system having been (ful)filled with competence as signified by licensure.

Medical communities in individual countries have developed a system for ensuring that this state is maintained by licensed practitioners. In Canada, MainCert is the Royal College's system for documenting maintenance of competence, which since 2001 has required, for ongoing fellowship certification, evidence of learning efforts in six identified areas (Royal College of Physicians and Surgeons of Canada 2007). In the United States, the American Board of Medical Specialties (ABMS) adopted in 2000 a requirement that each of its twenty-four member boards develop specific mechanisms for implementing a maintenance of competence (MOC) process. In both countries, the rationale for MOC is both quality and accountability. The ABMS explains that MOC constitutes an "[acknowledgment] of the growth and complexity of medical science, clinical care and the importance of the physician's relationship with the patient in delivering quality clinical outcomes"; a "proof that a physician has the practice-related knowledge to provide quality care in a particular specialty"; and "a professional response to the need for public accountability and transparency" (ABMS 1999). Interestingly, although its orientation is individualist in its provision of "focused learning based on individual practice needs," MOC has become a powerful surrogate for *system* quality. In the United States, owing in part to reduced malpractice claims associated with MOC participation, it is "recognized as an important quality marker by insurers, hospitals, quality and credentialing organizations as well as the federal government" (Pugh 2005).

Such programs reflect the premise that competence, once achieved, is not necessarily a permanent state; it can decline over time, but can be maintained through periodic influxes of learning. This premise, that the achieved *state* of *generic* competence is somewhat tenuous but maintainable through ongoing individual education activities, supports a CME industry of courses, guidelines, and audits designed to shore individual practitioners up against the threat of deteriorating knowledge or skill. In an online discussion thread, physicians aired this sense of threat, advising one another to take such MOC examinations as required by the American Board of Internal Medicine (ABIM) "as soon as possible and start studying as soon as possible, because if you wait nine years, you will be so out of shape that it will be impossible for you to catch up" (Student Doctor Network Forum 2010). As such comments imply, the MOC industry reinforces an individualist notion of competence both as something housed in the individual and, interestingly, as something that can deteriorate over time. In fact, nine years of practice is seen not as an additional source of competence-as-experience but as a threat to, or a potential dilution of, the competence-as-knowledge base acquired in residency.

Summary of the Individualist Way of Seeing

We should not be surprised that our way of seeing competence reflects the individualist orientation of the education system. This makes good sense, because the education system is predicated on the individualist orientation of the larger health care system, in which licensure, billing, and medicolegal accountability function on an individual practitioner basis (even in situations of collective decision making) (Sidhom and Poulsen 2006). And our health care system exists within a Western individualist society that pivots on the notion of the autonomous, conscious, rational human actor. As Burke put it, a god term manifests the "ultimate motive" of a community or context. Given that Western medicine is motivated by a depiction of the health care provider as an autonomous force (Gordon 1988), so too will the education of health care providers be motivated by similar values.

To summarize, then, competence *reflects* our individualist health care system and education culture. It *selects* for our attention individual learners and the knowledge, abilities, and values they possess in their heads, hands, and hearts. What, then, does it *deflect* our attention from? What blind spots does it produce? Here I return to the example I've encountered repeatedly in my field research on health care teams: competent individual professionals can—and do, with some regularity—combine to create an incompetent team. The conventional discourse of competence doesn't really help us grapple with this reality; it deflects our attention from this sticky educational and clinical problem. However, alternative ways of seeing competence are emerging that may help us address this.

An Emergent Way of Seeing

While the individualist approach is a dominant strain in past and current competence discourse in medical education, a new strain is coming into focus: a collectivist way of seeing competence. This emergence is motivated by growing attention in the social and organizational spheres to health care as a complex system, and to concerns about the quality of system performance in terms of issues such as teamwork and patient safety.

In this section, I draw together key theoretical premises that offer a basis for approaching competence as a collective, in addition to an individual, phenomenon. In tracing these premises, I suggest how they reframe the discourse to allow us to better articulate how teamwork is learned and enacted.

Premises Underpinning the Collectivist Discourse

This section will focus on the three key premises underpinning the collectivist discourse of competence in medical education:

1. Competence is achieved through participation in authentic situations.
2. Competence is distributed across a network of persons and artifacts.
3. Competence is a constantly evolving set of multiple, interconnected behaviors enacted in time and space.

Premise 1: Competence Is Achieved through Participation in Authentic Situations   *Collective competence* draws on social learning theory with its premise that knowledge is constructed through participation. Social learning theories attempt to move the focus beyond capturing, codifying, and documenting knowledge of individuals, and toward the ways through which knowledge is shared, discussed, and innovated in a collective setting. This focus is particularly appropriate in apprenticeship or work-based learning settings like medicine, where the emphasis on *participation* helps account for the relationships between experience, socialization, and identity construction.

A social approach to learning sees the learner not as the center, not as the agent who decides what knowledge to acquire in what settings, but as one part of a complex system of activity in which they must gain access to knowledge by interacting with artifacts, people, and processes. As Lave (1991) explains, "Learning, thinking, and knowing are relations among people engaged in activity *in, with and arising from the socially and culturally structured world* (67, emphasis in original). Reflecting a socio-cognitive perspective, Lave emphasizes the "relational interdependency of agent, and world, activity, meaning, cognition, learning and knowing" (ibid.). In these terms, the learning process is conceptualized as legitimate participation in social activities, such as the medical student's participation in the discussion of a patient's case on morning rounds with the internal medicine team. While teacher and learner influence what is learned, they do not entirely control it; learning is produced by the social interaction, which is shaped by the physical, social, and organizational context.

This sense of learning as situated, dynamic, and emergent, rather than generic and predetermined, is often referred to as "informal learning," a process through which the tacit knowledge of a community is developed, innovated, and shared (Bolhuis and Simons 2003; Eraut 2000; Hafferty

1998; Mittendorf et al. 2006). As Wenger (1998) points out, groups of people form communities of practice in which knowledge and expertise are deepened through ongoing interaction around authentic practices. In fact, Brown and Duguid (1996) argue that such tacit knowledge, essential for group functioning, can be externalized and spread only through social interaction. Such theories reclaim the terms "informal" and "tacit"; far from connoting a secondary or accidental form of knowledge, in the context of social and cultural learning theories these terms connote elemental, powerful forms of knowledge that underpin complex collaborative activities.

Such social learning theory is not just describing the development of individual competence through social interactions. There is a critical difference between learning in social interaction—where, for instance, participant A's knowledge is measurably improved as a consequence of the interaction experience—and learning collectively, which requires more than just individuals learning from others. Collective learning is visible when the *group's* shared knowledge and ability is influenced or improved as a consequence of their interaction. As Mittendorf et al. (2006) argue, new knowledge "has to be built...requiring intensive and laborious interaction among members of the organization and [the development of] a shared understanding or meaning about the knowledge that is created" (301). Researchers have begun to recognize how such intensive and laborious interaction is not only around the clinical work itself but also around new textual forms of *talking* that actually constitute the work (Iedema and Scheeres 2003). Through textual forms such as the briefing and debriefing routines increasingly common in the operating room, the interdisciplinary rounds that are emerging as routine on some inpatient wards, and the many variants of patient handover, teams are building collective knowledge about how to collaborate. Elaborating this insight, Bleakley, Bligh, and Browne (2011) describe a new, collective literacy emerging in the wake of interprofessional collaboration, which consists of the ability to talk about work roles, goals, and practices in ways that were not historically required. And with this new talk comes new social identities: Bleakley, Bligh, and Browne argue that "subjectivities or identities are not given, expressed and exercised, but are formed through the negotiations that go on within these new textualities of 'speaking out' about oneself in relation to a complex of Others" (89). Competence then, like identity, is not possessed by the individual but negotiated by the group, through work and talk.

Let's take an example from the operating room practice of briefing prior to a surgical procedure. In this case, let's say the surgeon leading the briefing does all the talking, without drawing on the knowledge and expertise of other team members. The anesthetist and circulating nurse allow the briefing to run its course, impatient with the tone but unwilling to interrupt. Clearly there is communicative incompetence here, but to locate it in one individual (or even within multiple individuals) is to miss the group's failure to have negotiated a team ethos in which ineffective briefing is redressed. The term "ethos" here reflects Bleakley, Bligh, and Browne's point that this is not simply a matter of knowledge, skills, or attitudes; it is a matter, fundamentally, of identity. Just as an effective briefing cannot be attributed to any single individual on the team, so too is an ineffective one a shared project. This leads us to the second theoretical premise underpinning a collective approach to competence: the importance of distributed cognition.

Premise 2: Competence Is Distributed across a Network of Persons and Artifacts   If we want to move from understanding learning and competence as statically based in individuals to seeing them as dynamically produced in situations, we require a different theory of how knowledge works. The concept of distributed cognition (Hutchins 1993) is a helpful place to start, as it takes as its unit of analysis a culturally constituted functional group rather than an individual mind. Distributed cognition sees collaborative work as "cognitive accomplishments" that "can be joint accomplishments, not attributable to any individual" (35). Such joint accomplishments emerge as information is propagated through a system in the form of representational states of mediating structures. It describes cognitive processes by tracing the movement of information through a system and characterizing the mechanisms of the system that carry out the performance, both on the individual and the group level.

Distributed cognition is a particularly useful concept for thinking about clinical training situations, in which knowledge is dynamic, learning is complex and uncertain, and information and rules are stored in technologies (e.g., computers) and in social traditions of clinical groups. As Bleakley and Bligh (2007, 80) argue, "Learning is largely a meta-process concerning legitimate access to situated (context-linked) and distributed knowing. This is not to deny the value of one's own store of knowledge, but to place this in the wider and more pressing context of learning how to learn or how to access knowledge." This is highly relevant to the context of team performance, in which competence includes knowing how to jointly produce knowledge, rather than how to individually reproduce information.

Hutchins and Klausen (1998) have used the theory of distributed cognition to explore the collective competence of the flight team working in an airline cockpit. Understanding the performance of the cockpit as a system requires both attention to the cognitive properties of the individual pilots and a new, larger unit of cognitive analysis that is composed of the pilots and their informational environment. This unit of analysis is termed a *system of distributed cognition*. For the system to be competent, to function effectively in a particular task, a number of features come into play. The key point is that "understanding the properties of individual cognition is only a small part of the effort to understand how complex human cognitive systems operate" (24). Let's again take the operating room as an example. Depending on the distribution of access to information and whether there exists a shared body of knowledge about the operation of the system, the operating room team may have shared expectations that serve as the basis of coordinated actions during the many tasks within a surgical procedure. The "coordination" made possible by distributed cognition is one representation of collective competence: shared knowledge helps produce shared mental representations of tasks, which assist shared expectations, which support coordinated actions.

How does this distribution of knowledge and coordination of actions happen, particularly for an interprofessional health care team where team members such as physicians, nurses, and therapists possess different knowledge and skills that they have developed in distinct training programs? Nonaka and Takeuchi (1995) point to the mobilization and conversion of tacit knowledge in collective learning situations, such that shared assumptions build up a context for effective prediction, and the capacity for coordination is formed. An intriguing example of such distributed cognition surrounds the phenomenon of silence on a team. Consider the following example (Lingard et al. 2009):

> The staff surgeon says loudly, without taking his eyes from the surgical field: "Almost certainly we're going to need a flexible sigmoidoscope and Dr. Black [a urologist]." The circulating nurse responds, using the staff surgeon's first name, "When, Larry?" There is no response from the staff

surgeon, who continues working. The nurse goes to call central processing to get the equipment sent up, after which she pages the urologist. (290)

Imagine that the urologist arrives just in time: she was, as it turned out,
needed immediately. How does the nurse know to page the urologist right
away, in the face of the silence that follows her question? How does the surgeon know that his silence will be interpreted as evidence that the situation
is urgent? It is not only the competence of the nurse, who may have noted
the critical situation that has been emerging in the procedure due to her
past experience. It is not merely the competence of the surgeon, who may
have worked with this nurse often enough to accurately predict that she
will correctly interpret his silence. It is the collective competence entailed
in the interaction of these: the nurse's and surgeon's shared knowledge—of
similar procedures, of one another's communication strategies, of the circumstances leading to a request for another specialist's presence in the operating room. This shared knowledge helps produce shared assumptions,
which build up a context for effective prediction, which supports coordinated actions. Of course, silence does not always signal shared knowledge
and distributed cognition: a lack of shared knowledge or shared mental
representations can lead to silence being misinterpreted. Imagine that the
urologist, Dr. Black, arrives long before she is actually required; in this
case, Dr. Black may be irritated at her wasted time, Larry may be frustrated that his request was misunderstood, and the circulating nurse may
be angry or embarrassed that she has mismanaged the flow of the procedure and the resources required to conduct it. But again, this incompetence
does not reside strictly within the individuals involved: it emerges from a
lack of collective learning, a failure to mobilize tacit knowledge in ways
that support distributed cognition across the group.

   This suggests that, as educators, we might turn our attention to assessing not only what individual team members know but their awareness of
what others know, their skill in the tacit and explicit forming of shared expectations, and their use of strategies to maximize coordination. The safety
literature has made great strides in articulating such capacities in ways that
support team performance assessment. For instance, Salas et al. (2007)
offer a framework for markers of "team cognition" consisting of three
markers of shared mental models ("closed loop communication," "mutual
performance monitoring," and "adaptive and supportive behavior") and

two markers of situation assessment ("problem identification and conceptualization" and "plan execution"). Each marker is specified into observable team behaviors. For instance, mutual performance monitoring, which is defined as the ability to "keep track of fellow team member's work while carrying out their own ... to ensure that everything is running as expected" (McIntyre and Salas 1995), is visible in behaviors such as "team members have an accurate understanding of their teammates' workload," "team members recognize when another team member makes a mistake," and "team members offer relevant knowledge before it is requested" (Salas et al. 2007). Such models of team cognition reflect the key notion of "coupling," the idea that parts of a system are not discrete, but rather that their connectedness is such that a change or weakness in one part of the system affects other parts and the performance of the whole.

When our attention is turned not to the *state* of individual team members but to their collective enactment of multiple threads of activity that in health care may be socio-spatially distributed among multiple organizational units, we are confronted with the third premise, which captures the instability of competence.

Premise 3: Competence Is a Constantly Evolving Set of Multiple, Interconnected Behaviors Enacted in Time and Space   Activity theory, arising from social learning theories, offers a language for characterizing the instability and impermanence of competence in the domain of teamwork. Originating in the work of Vygotsky (1978) and extended by Engeström (1987), activity theory offers the construct of an *activity system* to represent the complex interactions between individual human actors and the social, technological, and physical structures involved in their work. An activity theory framework considers individuals (*subjects*) as one aspect of a system that includes the tools (*artifacts*) they use to achieve goal-oriented outcomes (*objects*), while simultaneously being informed and influenced by both the norms (*rules*) of their social groups (*community*) and their conceptions of the appropriate organization and distribution of work (*division of labor*). For Engeström, these six points map an activity system in which all points are interconnected, so that a change anywhere in the system produces a ripple effect in all other elements. Using this way of thinking, an activity system like the operating room is inherently unstable, not only because the individual team members change during and across procedures, but because a variety of outcomes are at play at any time, a diverse array of social norms coexist both within and between the professional groups present for the activity, and there are ongoing, shifting tensions regarding the division of labor. In this regard, activity theory underscores the context dependency of competence, where a team may be competent at one point in time but not another, owing to shifts in any of Engeström's six factors (Cook and Yanow 1993; Sveiby 1997).

From a medical education perspective, this may seem an untenable proposition, for if competence is impermanent, if it must be negotiated anew whenever something in the activity system changes, then how can we ever certify any health care team as capable of safe practice? Engeström's theory of *knotworking* provides a way of modeling how teams manage such instability, how they can integrate their efforts in ways that produce competent performances in a continuous cycle in the face of complex and shifting systems. Knotworking is a form of discursive work organization that Engeström characterizes as "a movement of tying, untying and re-tying together seemingly separate threads of activity" (Engeström 2000, 972). When barriers to the progress of care halt the team's work and require their improvisation to move forward, these represent knotworking instances in the team activity system. For instance, if the clinical treatments enacted by cardiology and respirology produce conflicting outcomes for a patient, or when a family's expectations for discharge diverge from others' expectations, teams must respond to these evolutions in the activity system in order to keep the care plan on track. Key features of knotworking are its shifting locus of initiative/control and its lack of fixed end point—at its essence, the phenomenon is adaptive, continuous, and distributed across time and space. The construct holds promise for improved understanding of the amorphous process that is distributed, collaborative care, in which health providers separated by time and space continuously negotiate values, meanings, and care plans throughout a patient's trajectory. Attention to knotworking practices may improve our understanding of fissures, bridges, and innovations in the distributed network of care, and inform our efforts to redesign them for improved quality.

Summary of the Collectivist Way of Seeing

The collectivist approach emerges at a time when health care is increasingly understood as a complex system, rather than a dyadic relationship between a provider and a patient. It is resonant with a movement to recognize the role of collaborative practice in quality health care delivery. And it reflects theories of social learning and distributed cognition, which emphasize the joint construction of meaning, identity, and work. As a way of seeing, the collectivist approach is also a way of not seeing: it *reflects* a systems orientation and an acceptance of the instability of performance, *selecting* for our attention joint accomplishments and social negotiations, while *deflecting* our attention from individual agency, memory, and expertise.

Implications of Integrating Both Discourses

This chapter has described two discourses of—or *ways of seeing*—competence in medical education. The individualist discourse approaches competence as an individual possession that is stable and context-free, while the collectivist discourse approaches competence as a distributed capacity that is evolving and based in situations. While I have elaborated the critical differences between these two discourses, my intent is not to set up a binary opposition between them: the collectivist discourse is not a "solution" to the individualist discourse. Rather, each discourse selects and deflects, drawing our attention to some aspects of competence and leaving other aspects unaddressed. And each discourse emerges from a set of theoretical constructs and values that shape educators' sense of what to teach and what to assess in medicine. Thus, I'm not proposing *collective competence* as a replacement god term.

What I am proposing is that an appreciation of both discourses could lead health professional educators to a better language for describing and assessing competence in this era of increasing emphasis on teamwork. The idea that a multidimensional understanding of education is necessary to capture its complexity is not new. In fact, over a decade ago, a similar argument underpinned Sfard's (1998) description of two learning metaphors: *acquisition* and *participation*. She argued that the acquisition metaphor, which approaches learning as the acquisition of knowledge, skills, attributes, values, and competencies, reinforces learning as an individual process. She noted, as I have earlier in this chapter, that this metaphor is so deeply embedded in our thinking that we scarcely notice it until other metaphors begin to emerge. In contrast, the metaphor of participation views learning not as something to be acquired or achieved; rather, participation *is* learning and, consequently, learning (like participation) is viewed as a continuous process. Furthermore, whereas acquisition implies that knowledge can be transferred across situations, participation sees learning as inextricably tied to its context. Sfard cautions that it is probably not in learners' interest to adopt just one metaphor. Instead we need to think about pedagogical approaches that support both.

Since discourses (and metaphors) are not sequential but overlapping—responsive to diverse needs and reflective of competing values—I propose that we consider how a collectivist discourse of competence might interact with, and be implemented alongside, our dominant, individualist one. To demonstrate the different insights made possible by these two discourses, let's consider the following anecdote from "one morning in the operating room," which is derived from my field research in operating rooms:

> During a liver resection, the surgeon requests more sponges due to heavy bleeding. She asks the anesthetist what the central venous pressure (CVP) is.
>
> "Fifteen," he replies.
>
> She raises her head: "What? Fifteen? No wonder we've got all this bleeding." Shakes her head, saying to the resident, "It should be kept less than 5 when we're transecting the liver. We're going to have to try and hurry this up."
>
> Surgeon asks anesthetist: "Can you lower the CVP? It will help the blood loss by reducing the backpressure from the hepatic veins."
>
> Anesthetist: "Yes, but he won't tolerate a CVP less than 5. He needs a high preload to maintain output."
>
> Surgeon: "If you don't lower it, he's going to lose a lot of blood and that won't be pretty either!"

During liver surgery, the surgeon will prefer to maintain a low central venous pressure (CVP). Particularly at the point of cutting through the liver, the surgeon prefers the CVP to be less than 5 because the decreased pressure in the veins decreases bleeding and blood loss. If the anesthetist commonly works on liver cases, or if the team discusses concerns about bleeding before the case, then they will have shared expectations regarding the CVP at the point of resection and their actions will be coordinated around that particular moment and task. This coordination is critical, as it takes some time to decrease the CVP, which requires prediction and coordination on the part of the anesthetist to time the decrease appropriately.

From an individualist way of seeing, we would ask particular questions in our attempt to understand the underpinnings of this exchange. Focused on individual skills, knowledge, and attitudes, we might ask questions such as:

- What does the anesthetist know? Is he familiar with liver resection procedures or does he usually work in another surgical service? What is his level of expertise? Is he a staff person, fellow, or resident?
- What does the surgeon know? Is she familiar with—or does she recall at this moment—the patient's heart condition? Does she understand the timing issues associated with lowering the CVP? Is she familiar with this anesthetist's approach? What kind of a communicator is she?

There are advantages to this way of seeing the situation. It can reveal individual areas that need improvement, such as the surgeon's lack of understanding of the timing issues associated with lowering the CVP. And this way of seeing can foster a sense of individual responsibility, because attention is focused on each individual actor's knowledge and skill. The key disadvantage of the individualist way of seeing is that, as the dominant discourse, it may carry the assumption that individual strengths and weaknesses are the only source of strength and weakness on the team. This assumption produces beliefs such as: "If every person in the room was at the top of their game, then this team would work just fine" and "You do your job, I'll do mine, and we'll have a smooth morning." Such beliefs may blind team members and educators to other sources of competence and incompetence on the team, making system-wide improvements difficult.

A collectivist way of seeing the CVP anecdote would draw our attention to other factors. We might ask whether the team members have shared knowledge about the preference for a CVP less than 5 during resection to limit blood loss, because if this shared knowledge does not exist, then shared expectations cannot exist either. If the surgeon falsely assumes shared expectations and the anesthetist does not share the goal of bringing the CVP down, then the surgeon may not notice until the onset of heavy bleeding; by then it is too late, as the CVP cannot be decreased instantaneously to correct the bleeding problem during resection. And since lowered CVP is not automatically appropriate for all patients (some will not tolerate a low CVP because of certain heart conditions), the team must establish whether the strategy of lowered CVP is defensible for this patient with a heart condition. The team must collectively establish the knowledge about the patient and the CVP/bleeding issue in order to produce shared expectations required for coordinated action.

These are some of the questions we might ask from the perspective of collective competence:

- What is the access to information across the group? Are team members aware of what others know and don't know about this particular patient and this particular procedure? Are team members aware of what others expect?
- What are the similarities and differences in team members' perceptions of the situation? Do they share a perception of the patient's status, the relative advantage of lowered CVP, and the nature of an emergency?
- What are their respective roles in relation to decisions about the ideal CVP level for a patient, and do they share an understanding of how that decision should be negotiated?

These questions reflect a concern with the team's shared mental model. A case like this one reminds us that shared mental models can be formal and institutionalized at a macro level, or informal and local. An iconic example at the macro level is the crew resource management approach in aviation, which allows for interchangeability of players because there is an institutionalized mental model that governs how team members will respond in critical situations. In fact, in this team culture interchangeability is encouraged, in part so that this shared mental model is not weakened by partners becoming familiar enough with each other to negotiate local adaptations of it. In most health care settings, if shared mental models exist they are largely informal and negotiated through the ongoing interactions of a familiar team. However, in the absence of both team stability and an institutionalized, formal model that makes members interchangeable, such negotiations may be required at a burdensome rate. Worse still, different health care professions (say, in the case of our operating room anecdote, anesthesia and surgery) may possess different formal or informal mental models that shape their expectations of how events should unfold at any point in the procedure. If these models have not been institutionally negotiated across the professions, then individual negotiations are required to allow flexibility and explicit cross-checking; however, in a moment of urgency, like the CVP exchange, they may be difficult to successfully manage.

The advantage of the collectivist way of seeing is that it draws attention to all potential fault lines in a team of competent individuals, including issues such as shared expectations and role clarity. With reference to aviation teams, Hutchins and Klausen (1998, 16) put it this way: "The question should not be whether a particular pilot is performing well, but whether or not the *system* that is composed of the pilot, co-pilot and the technology of the cockpit is performing well. It is the performance of that system, not the skills of any individual pilot, that determines whether you live or die." A comprehensive analysis of the competence of this operating room team performance would combine both the individualist and the collectivist way of seeing, attending broadly to the entire activity system of the operating room, including

- the cognitive properties of individuals (what does the surgeon know? the anesthetist? the nurse?);
- the physical properties of tools in the environment that represent knowledge and action (what is recorded on the paper chart? how is information organized in the computer? what equipment is available? do the nurse and surgeon have access to the same information?);
- the interactions of meta-representations held by team members (what are the similarities and differences in how the surgeon and anesthetist perceive the patient's status, the goal of the procedure, and the nature of an "emergency"?).

From an analytical perspective, employing both ways of seeing competence is powerful and can usefully open up a number of areas of inquiry in health professions education that are currently limited to an individualist way of seeing. Take the domain of professionalism, for example. In the past decade, professionalism research has focused on individual dimensions of this phenomenon, exploring how medical students respond to professional dilemmas (Ginsburg, Regehr, and Lingard 2003), how professional values change over the course of a student's training (Satterwhite, Satterwhite, and Enarson 2000), or how faculty approach the assessment of a student's professionalism (Ginsburg, Regehr, and Lingard 2004). Yet we all recognize that students make and enact their professional decisions in social contexts. Incorporating a collectivist way of seeing would enrich our research in this area, positioning us to ask the following sorts of questions:

- By what process do students negotiate their individual professional ethos with a clinical team's collective professional ethos?

- When there is incongruity between individual and collective professional ethos, what happens?
- Do students accommodate their individual values to the team's, or does a student sometimes sway the team's professional decision?

Such scenarios present a rich opportunity to explore the mutual influences of individual and collective competence, toward a better understanding of the complexity of their interrelationship.

There is strong analytical value to conceptualizing health professional education questions using both discourses of competence. But what about practical value? Can the two discourses coexist given the different theories and values underpinning them? Take the practicalities of assessment, for example. Individualist discourse reflects traditional values (such as autonomy), supports key agendas (such as licensure), and is facilitated by a vast assessment infrastructure (Hodges 2006). By contrast, collectivist discourse reflects new values such as systems approach, supports emerging agendas such as collaborative practice, and would require a new assessment infrastructure for measuring team performance. Incorporating a collectivist discourse will change the kinds of expressions that can be made about competence: we will have to shift from talking just about *competent practitioners* to talking also about *competent performances* of teams. We will not be able to think along the lines of competent teams per se, since a team's competent performance in one situation may not necessarily predict its competent performance in another situation. We will have to attend to situation a great deal more than we currently do, in both our teaching (e.g., teaching the individual skills and collective ethos of situational assessment and mutual performance monitoring) and in our development of assessment tools and goals. However, this shift in perspective to include a collectivist way of seeing may create a deep tension between our educational and evaluative activities and the core values of psychometric assessment. If we accept the premises that competence is developed in participation, that it is tied to context, and that it is unstable, then how can we create objective, valid, and reliable measurement instruments to capture this emerging, fluid, and impermanent phenomenon? Professional organizations will still face the challenge of certifying that those delivering health care have sufficient expertise to practice safely and effectively. How can a collectivist discourse of competence address this need?

Interestingly, this challenge is already being faced to some extent, with the acknowledgment of the difficulties of reliable and valid measurement of the core competencies. Some in the debate have argued that a universal definition of any of the competencies is impossible because each is inextricably socially located. As McGaghie et al. (1978, 23) assert, "The definition of medical competence is bound to local political, social, and economic circumstances, to health needs, to the availability of resources, and to the structure of the health care system. Thus any effort to find a universal definition of competence will inevitably fail." Others recognize that the attempt to develop reliable and valid assessment measures for the competencies has been largely unsuccessful. As Lurie, Mooney, and Lyness (2009) have reported in a review, the only ACGME competency for which proven measurement tools exist is that of medical knowledge— the competency most readily conceptualized as *possessed* by an individual practitioner. Regardless of this poor progress in the assessment of the competencies, however, Lurie, Mooney, and Lyness stand by them as articulated:

> This is not because the general competencies are, in any sense, "incorrect"; rather, it is a reflection of the Outcome Project's assumption that the general competencies, once defined, would reveal themselves in a straightforward fashion through measurement. It will remain a challenge to develop objective measures that correspond neatly to these generalized educational constructs. In addition to disagreements over theoretical issues, measurement of actual human behaviors is subject to a host of non-theoretical biases and technical challenges, including the well-known psychometric problems of method variance, observer biases, expectation and contextual effects, logistical constraints, and random error. (307)

One wonders whether it is the collectivist aspects of the other core competencies that defy our traditional psychometric assessment techniques. The review by Lurie, Mooney, and Lyness is an embodiment of the individualist discourse of competence and so they do not explicitly explore the idea that the individualist approach to the core competencies may be part of the problem; that is, that we have taken a collectivist phenomenon, named it using individualist language, and accordingly applied individualist assessment theories to little effect. They do, however, point to an interesting development suggestive of this logic, as they consider "the two newer

ACGME competencies: systems-based practice (SBP) and problem-based learning and improvement (PBLI)":

> SBP and PBLI...are viewed by many authors as representing aspects of health systems and teams rather than those of particular individuals. Thus, it is possible that environmental variables may exert significant influence on trainees' behaviors surrounding these competences. It is possible, for instance, that a trainee with relatively good understanding of systems-based issues may nonetheless seem to perform poorly when placed in a practice environment that hinders good communication among caregivers. Further refinements of the operational definitions of these competencies should include measures of health systems in addition to any measures of individuals. (307)

This chapter presents a language for articulating two ways of seeing competence—an individualist approach that is pervasive, tacit, and normalized in health professional education, and a collectivist approach that is emergent and directs our attention to features of competence necessary for conceptualizing it in the context of teamwork. Understanding that our notion of competence *is constructed,* that it *selects* and *deflects* our attention, may put us in the position to grapple in new ways with the difficulties Lurie, Mooney, and Lyness outline. Further, seeing competence as constructed, and recognizing the potential for multiple constructions, is a necessary first step in guarding against naive acceptance that "competence is competence is competence." As Burke (1952) suggests, the danger with god terms is that, through repeated use and familiarity, they become suggestive of a natural, universal, and inevitable order of reality. Teasing apart the current discourse of competence is an exercise in making it unfamiliar, excavating the motivations that underpin it, and opening space for an adaptive and flexible discourse of competence that positions us to make new advances in research and practice.

PERTURBATIONS

The Central Role of Emotional Competence in Medical Training

Nancy McNaughton and Vicki LeBlanc

In this chapter we examine the role of emotion as an integral, and often underappreciated, component of competency in the health professions from different scientific perspectives and discuss the implications for health professional training and practice.

Within the health professions, emotion sits uneasily at the intersection between objective scientific fact and subjective humanistic values as a site of productive contestation. It is widely acknowledged as a core element of professional values, attitudes, and beliefs, as well as of humanistic approaches to professional activities—counseling, patient management, and communication. It is also recognized as an essential aspect of professional well-being and patient satisfaction. Emotion is, however, only peripherally embedded in our discussions of learning, acquisition of knowledge and skills, and the development of expertise. Unexamined notions and naive understanding about emotion—how it works, what it consists of, how it shapes practice and thought—have practical implications.

As they relate to competency, ideas about emotion in health professional education activate particular assumptions that produce and reproduce professional expectations about emotion in practice. These ideas are embedded in both formal and informal curricular structures and in professional documents, producing effects on practice and policy related to professionalism and competency. Theories about emotion range along a continuum from purely physiological at one end to wholly sociocultural at the other. Along this continuum, certain views predominate within health professional education with repercussions for professional training and practice. For instance, one perspective suggests that emotion is an interaction of subjective and physiological processes through which cognitive abilities are shaped, particularly attention, memory, and decision making. In this framework, information about emotions as physiological processes can occur through measures of hormones in the saliva. Another perspective suggests that emotion is also socially and culturally constructed, focusing on interactions between individuals and society more than on our emotions' internal mechanisms. As such, our epistemological lenses direct our focus as researchers to ask different questions about emotion, which in turn lead to different expectations about emotional competency in professional practice.

It is our suggestion that the many views and approaches to the study of emotion in the health professions contribute to an enriched understanding about emotion in practice, while also expanding our ability as researchers and educators to appreciate emotion as the multidimensional topic that it is.

In the following sections we provide definitions of emotion from the domains of science and social science, followed by discussions of the integral role that emotion plays in health professional practice both at the individual and sociocultural level. Within these discussions, we examine how different assumptions are—or are not—embedded in our conceptualizations of competence in health professions. We conclude with some thoughts on the risks of incomplete or naive understandings about emotion with regard to health professional training and practice, and offer several possible paths to embedding more nuanced thinking about emotions into our conceptualizations of health professional competence.

Assumptions about Emotions in the Health Professions

Emotion Is the Opposite of Reason

Traditionally, emotion has been seen as separate from rationality—on the other side of the Cartesian divide. Cartesian dualities, such as mind/body and reason/emotion, are central to a dominant Western viewpoint. They are perpetuated in part by the effects of scientific and technological developments that find "emotion as a corruption of reason that needs to be transcended" (Williams 2001, xvi). Williams suggests that reason is regarded as indispensable for the acquisition of truth. Within clinical practice, reason is valued as one of the most important ingredients for competent practice in the form of good, objective decisions. In contrast, emotions are generally perceived as dangerous, unpredictable, beyond our control, and in need of managing. Emotion is contrasted with, and less valued than, rationality.

As an example, a significant body of research has been devoted to understanding the development of expertise, both in terms of how experienced clinicians organize information in their minds and in terms of their clinical reasoning and decision making (Eva 2005). Important insights into the reasoning strategies of health professionals have been garnered. We have strong evidence to suggest that when faced with straightforward clinical scenarios, clinicians tend to engage in automatic processing that makes use of heuristics, and when they are faced with challenging scenarios, they are more likely to engage in deliberate, effortful processing (Chapter 7). We also have gained significant insights into how different approaches to teaching clinical concepts can lead to better reasoning and guard one from biasing information (Eva et al. 2007). However, the focus of this domain of research has been solely on the cognitive, or rational, aspect of decision making. The role that emotion plays in clinical reasoning and decision making has not been explored in health professions. Furthermore, none of this research has examined how sociocultural norms related to emotion may influence the manifestations of emotion in professional practice.

Emotions Are Dangerous

Within clinical training and practice, both the experience and expression of emotion are deemed problematic except in their positive guise as altruism and empathy. "The hierarchy between emotion and thought/reason gets displaced into a hierarchy between emotions: some emotions are elevated as signs of cultivation, whilst others remain lower as signs of weakness" (Ahmed 2004, 2). The suggestion seems to be that some emotions are good while others are bad, with the negative ones needing to be dispatched while preserving the positive. Whether good or bad, emotions are regarded as having a life of their own and being in the way, overwhelming our reason and possibly leading to dangerous decisions and actions. Common phrases such as "I lost my head" and "I need to get a grip" reflect this view of emotions. A similar notion is that emotions occur like naturalized weather patterns (Boler 1999, 205). In this view, it is not emotions themselves—either positive or negative—that are troublesome, but rather their occurrence, which is unpredictable and unstoppable. Like naturalized weather patterns, emotions are ever present and almost constantly in flux. Just as it would be bad to never have rain because of the essential role it plays for all forms of life, it would be detrimental to humans and society to attempt to eliminate emotions such as fear, anger, and so forth. So rather than pathologizing the emotions themselves, such a view holds that it is the invisibility and seeming unpredictability of physiological processes that are problematic.

That health care professionals need to make objective and rational decisions is not in dispute. However, the important role that emotion plays in attention, memory, decision-making processes, and creative problem solving is becoming clearer with recent research in the cognitive and neurosciences, as will be discussed further in this chapter.

Furthermore, ideas about emotions have real effects on professional training and practice. They are a social and cultural phenomenon as much as physiological and psychological. Emotion and its expression are negotiated according to social and cultural criteria. Not everyone has the same permission to express themselves emotionally in different social contexts. In addition, certain expressions of emotion are considered professionally inappropriate and may be read as signs of trouble producing regulatory classifications such as "the disruptive doctor" (Policy Statement 4–07 College of Physicians and Surgeons of Ontario).

In the health professions, we have adopted a Darwinian model of emotions, which suggests that emotions are not only beneath us but are part of our prehistory as signs of an earlier, more primitive time. In this adoption, emotion and reason are set up in opposition to each other with emotion figured as less-valued, malleable raw material. "The story of evolution is narrated not only as the story of the triumph of reason, but of the ability to control emotions, and to experience the 'appropriate' emotions at different times and places" (Elias 1978).

Definitions of Emotions

As an object of study, emotion is notoriously difficult to delineate, with little agreement between professions or even within disciplines about what it is. It is variously described as physiologically determined (Damasio 1994; Darwin 1872; LeDoux 1996), internally experienced and natural (Gardner 1985; Goleman 1995), a component of reason (Aristotle 1961; Hume 1711–1776; Lazarus 1991; Spencer 1862), a medium for the transmission of sociocultural values and/or the result of sociocultural practices (Hall 1997; Hochschild 2003; Kemper 1993; Lutz and Abu-Lughod 1990), a performance (Bhaba 1987; Butler 2005; Foucault 1980), or central to aesthetic and moral experience (Greene 1973; Noddings 1984; Nussbaum 1996). Each of these views constructs emotion in ways that make certain actions and roles possible while constraining others. Given that the health professions are constituted by science, social science, and the humanities, each of these views can inform discussions about the place of varying constructions of emotion with respect to health care competencies. For an effective discussion of emotions, however, it is important to contextualize them within one's discourse, or else they risk creating more ambiguity than clarity (Gendron and Barrett 2009).

Emotions at the Neurological Level

One neuroscience approach has proposed that emotions within the individual can occur without the subjective experience of feelings (Naqvi, Shiv, and Bechara 2006). This approach explores how the brain processes emotional information. While unconscious processes can lead to conscious experiences of feelings, this is not always the case. Emotions can be a series of physiological or neuronal responses to situations that inform the organism about situations that are desired or undesired (Damasio1994). Within the broad field of emotion studies, these can also be labeled "sensations."

An example of the distinction between conscious subjective and unconscious physiological manifestation of emotions can be found in the research on stress. Stress responses can manifest themselves with the consciously experienced feelings of anxiety. Yet they can also manifest themselves in physiological activation of the brain's stress response system, which leads to the release of the stress hormone cortisol. While anxiety and cortisol responses often occur together, individuals can have physiological cortisol responses in the absence of experiencing increases in anxiety. Furthermore, the two can have different effects on thought and behavior (Regehr et al. 2008).

Emotions at a Cognitive Level

Emotions can also be understood as the more familiar conscious subjective experience of feelings or moods—feeling anxious, happy, or frustrated—and form an integral part of cognitive function (Izard 2009). As well, cognitive activities (functions) can contribute to the elicitation of emotions. Many models of emotion from this perspective suggest that emotions are not merely triggered by objects and situations in reflexive or habitual ways (Gendron and Barrett 2009), but also arise from the meaningful interpretation of objects and situations by the individual: an emotion emerges when a person's internal state is understood in some way as related to or caused by the situation. Research in this domain (Harvey et al. 2010; LeBlanc et al. 2010) is concerned with the process by which appraisals lead to the elicitation of emotions, as well as how emotions interact with cognitive functions to influence how we perceive, pay attention to, remember information from, and make decisions about the world around us in various emotional or mood states.

Emotion at the Sociocultural Level

Emotion is seen to be constructed in interaction between people with emotions themselves arising as socially determined effects within a sociocultural framing. It is still accepted as physiological, internal to the individual, and valuable as a form of cognition in appraising and interpreting our environment. However, it is also envisioned as an effect of social and cultural forces (Ahmed 2004; Boler 1999; Solomon 2007) and thus also responsible for creating normative understandings about appropriate behaviors, roles, and activities. In other words, emotion may act as a social force.

Sociocultural approaches to emotion range from cognitive behavioral to social performative. Those who adopt behavioral methods treat emotion as part of an observable skill set that is amenable to educative processes like practice or self-reflection. For example, Aristotle's famous statement "Anyone can become angry—that is easy. But to be angry with the right person, to the right degree, at the right time, for the right purpose and in the right way—this is not easy" (cited in Goleman 1995, xix) suggests that emotions such as anger are tied to an individual's social investments that are performed in relation to social status. Emotions in this respect are skills that can be used to gain status, as much as attributes of individual biology, and are changeable and can be practiced and improved. More radical social theories of emotion frame them as a circulating force, a medium of exchange, or a form of labor (Ahmed 2004; Boler 1999; Hochschild 2003), and as such explore emotion's political and cultural effects. Many critical social theorists bypass questions about the effect of emotion on individual behavior to focus on its role in shaping power relations, posing questions such as who decides which emotions are appropriate in different contexts? How are inappropriate emotions policed?

According to this viewpoint, the words used to describe emotions are not simply names for "emotion entities," preexisting things with coherent characteristics. Rather, these words are themselves actions or ideological practices "that serve specific purposes in the process of creating and negotiating reality" (Lutz and Abu-Lughod 1990, 4). Language used to speak about emotion within a social situation is seen to constitute meaning and experience as much as label it. Social scientists do not deny the physiological and psychological explanations of emotion and our experience of it. Rather, they focus their attention on the effects that different conceptions of emotion have in shaping professional, organizational, and personal life.

The Role of Emotions in Individual and Social Life

In the following sections we will elaborate on how various schools of thought—the neuronal, the cognitive, and the sociocultural—can inform our thinking about the integral role of emotion in both individual and social functions. These arguments will then be used to inform our discussion regarding their significance for our understanding of competency in the health professions.

A Neuroscience Perspective

In much of the research on human thought and emotions, it was long assumed that the emotional groundings of human behavior are separate from the more rational and superior groundings of thought (Gros 2010). Early research into the site of emotions in the brain led to the proposal that emotions could be found in the limbic system, a discrete network of primitive structures in the brain between the neocortex (the seat of cognitive and learning capacities) and the brain stem (responsible for basics of life maintenance such as breathing, heartbeat, and blood pressure). This limbic system perspective viewed emotions as residing in a part of the brain that was, from an evolutionary perspective, older and less evolved. The more evolved part of the brain, the neocortex, was seen as responsible for the cognitive functions that distinguish humans from less evolved animals: reasoning, decision making, anticipation, and planning. The result of this conceptualization of emotions as being localized in the older, more reptilian, part of the brain was the devaluation of emotions as primitive and antithetical to reason and higher order cognition.

Several advances in neuroscience have challenged the concept that emotions and cognitive functions are processed in separate parts of the brain. First, research has revealed that the "newer" and "reptilian" parts of the brain do not differ from each other as much as originally believed (Damasio 1994). Second, input from the subcortical emotional systems into the cognitive systems is stronger than input from the cognitive systems to the emotional ones, suggesting a primacy for emotional processing over cognitive processing. Finally, structures believed to be part of the "emotional" limbic system (e.g., the hippocampus) are found to have a very active involvement in cognitive processes (e.g., memory), and structures believed to be responsible for cognitive functions are found to have an active role in processing emotional information. Emerging from this work is a picture of emotions as actively involved in many areas of the human brain and tightly interwoven with structures of memory, attention, and decision making (Damasio 1994). There is growing recognition, from a number of domains, that emotions have a function that is indispensable to human cognitive processes (Gros 2010). Without them, humans are incapable of functioning. Emotion and cognition not only interact in the brain but are often integrated such that they jointly contribute to behavior (Pessoa 2008). As demonstrated by Damasio, "when emotion is entirely left out of the reasoning picture ... reason turns out to be even more flawed than when emotion plays bad tricks on our decisions" (Damasio 1994, xii). Some of the more powerful evidence against the separation of emotion and cognition comes from studies looking at the roles of the amygdala and the prefrontal cortex.

The amygdala is one of the brain structures thought to be the most important for the processing of emotional information (LeDoux 1996; Phelps 2006). It plays an integral role in processing fear information, as well as in processing social cues and faces, particularly when they are emotional in nature. Damage to the amygdala impairs the ability to process emotional facial expressions. In addition, individuals with damage to their amygdala do not show the enhanced memory for the emotional aspects of a story that is observed in normal individuals (Adolphs, Tranel, and Buchanan 2005; Phelps 2006). These findings from brain-damaged patients are supported by brain imaging research. For example, several brain imaging studies, using PET scans and fMRIs, showed brain activation in the amygdala when individuals were presented with emotional faces, even when those faces were presented so rapidly that the individuals were not aware of them (Dalgleish 2004; Morris et al. 2001; Whalen et al. 1998). Additionally, PET scan studies show that the amount of activation of the amygdala when individuals are first presented with emotional information predicts the accuracy of recall of that information several weeks later (Kensinger 2009). Put together, this body of literature suggests that the amygdala, which was historically believed to be involved solely in the processing of emotions, also plays an important role in cognitive functions, particularly the processing and interpretation of emotional social information and memory of emotional information.

Conversely, the prefrontal cortex, which had historically been thought to be responsible solely for the planning of behavior, decision making, and social behavior, has been shown to also have a role in emotions (Dalgleish 2004). One of the more famous cases that supports this role is that of Phineas Gage, a construction worker who suffered damage to his prefrontal cortex when a railway explosion propelled a one-meter-long iron rod straight through his head, entering just below the eye socket and exiting through the top of his head. As a result of this accident, Gage, who had previously been an amiable and reliable man, became irreverent, impatient, quick to anger, and unreliable.

Subsequent research with individuals with damage to the prefrontal cortex showed that they exhibit decision-making patterns that are detrimental to their well-being (Dalgleish 2004; Damasio 1994). Despite having intact intellectual and problem-solving abilities, these individuals consistently make decisions that lead to financial, social-status, and interpersonal losses. They appear unable to learn from their mistakes and repeatedly engage in decisions that lead to negative consequences. Furthermore, these individuals have flat affects and are impaired in their ability to react to emotional situations. These findings suggest that the patients with damage to the ventromedial prefrontal cortex are unable to use their emotions as an aid to decision making, particularly when the outcomes of the decision are uncertain (Bechara et al. 1994; Bechara, Tranel, and Damasio 2000).

A leading hypothesis to emerge from this body of work, the somatic marker hypothesis, suggests that emotions, in the form of bodily states, can bias decision making toward choices that will maximize the likelihood of reward and minimize the likelihood of punishment (Damasio 1994, 1997; Damasio, Everitt, and Bishop 1996). Somatic markers are physiological reactions that tag previous events that had an emotional outcome. They provide a signal when individuals are faced with a current situation that is similar to one that had emotion-related consequences in the past. These markers influence individuals in situations of uncertainty, where decisions need to be made on the basis of the emotional properties of the present situation. As such, emotions can represent the unconscious assessment of bodily sensations and physical changes, and these motivate and direct action or thinking (Damasio 1994, 1997; Damasio, Everitt, and Bishop 1996). They allow decisions to be made when a logical analysis of the available choices is insufficient.

In the health professions, there is very little integration of these concepts into our understanding of competency. There is also very little discussion not only of the role of emotions but also of the neural and physiological underpinning of thought and behavior. One exception is in the study of stress and physiological arousal, a recent domain of inquiry. Researchers who are interested in the role of stress and arousal in performance and learning have been paying close attention to the contributions of activation of the hypothalamic-pituitary-adrenal axis (and the ensuing release of the stress hormone cortisol) and of the sympathetic nervous system arousal (and the ensuing increase in heart rate) on performance in high acuity domains (Arora et al. 2010; Harvey et al. 2011; LeBlanc et al. 2010; Wetzel et al. 2010). In addition, researchers are seeking to better understand the factors that lead to manifestations of physiological stress and arousal in high pressure domains (Harvey et al. 2010), as well as the impact of various educational approaches on physiological stress responses of trainees (Arora et al. 2011; Bong et al. 2010).

A Cognitive Perspective

The neuroscience literature described above reveals how brain structures previously thought to solely process emotional information actually play an important role in cognitive functions, and that regions previously thought to process cognitive information also process emotional information used in making decisions when faced with uncertainty. This literature also shows that when the ability to process emotional information is impaired through brain injury, performance on cognitive tasks is impaired. Together, this body of literature challenges the commonly held assumption about the separation of emotion from cognition in the brain. As described below, research from cognitive sciences also reveals that subjectively experienced emotions and feelings can play an important role in shaping cognitive processes, such as attention, perception, memory, and decision making.

Attention and perception are the first stages in processing information. Factors that influence these will also influence subsequent stages of processing, including memory and reasoning. There is a growing body of literature showing that emotions play an important role in our ability to attend to and process the world around us. Further discussion of cognitive theories related to attention and its allocation can be found in chapter 7 of this volume, by Leung, Epstein, and Moulton. People show enhanced perception for emotionally significant information, and their interpretation of events tends to reflect their current emotional state. They demonstrate a more rapid detection of, and a preference for, emotionally congruent information such as facial expressions (Dolan 2002; Nabi 2003; Niedenthal and Setterlund 1994). Anxiety, even when mild, is associated with an increased likelihood of interpreting ambiguous stimuli (facial expressions, social situations, heard homophones) as threatening (Blanchette and Richards 2003; Richards et al. 2002). In fact, it is difficult to disengage attention from the emotional qualities of a stimulus, particularly negatively valenced ones (Phelps 2006).

Emotion also plays an important role in memory function. Most readers will be familiar with the experience of encountering events that were so emotionally charged as to become indelibly marked in memory, whether they are personal events such as when a loved one is injured or public events such as the *Challenger* explosion or the events of September 11. The literature does support this phenomenon, demonstrating that emotions can enhance memory for some details of an experience. Specifically, memory enhancements for emotionally arousing events will occur for those details that arouse the emotions. Memory for more peripheral details will not be enhanced, and oftentimes can be impaired (Kensinger 2009). This occurs partly because of the attentional effects of emotions described above; information that elicits emotions is more likely to be attended to, and thus is more likely to be encoded in memory. Improved memory also occurs due to enhanced consolidation, the process by which memories are turned into stable and lasting representations (Kensinger 2009). These memory enhancements appear to be stronger for negative events than for positive events. In contrast to the facilitating effects of emotions on memory encoding and consolidation, emotions can impair the recall of previously learned information, such as formulas for drug dosage calculations (LeBlanc et al. 2005).

Emotions also appear to have an impact on individuals' decision-making process. Both because they serve an information function (a negative mood is informative of a problematic situation that needs to be addressed) and because they can influence what information is attended to in a particular situation, emotions can have an important effect on decision making. For example, sad individuals are biased toward options that present high risks and the possibility of high reward. In contrast, individuals who are anxious are biased toward low-risk options that also present low rewards (Raghunathan and Pham 1999). A very common finding in the "regret research" is the *action effect,* where negative outcomes resulting from action are found to lead to regret more often than do the same outcomes achieved through inaction. However, when decisions are made following a negative outcome, an *inaction effect* can occur. That is, after a negative outcome, inaction can lead to more regret than action does if a second negative outcome occurs (Zeelenberg et al. 2002). Thus, the "regret" individuals feel because they previously failed to accurately predict risk of harm may cause them to over- or underestimate risk in a new situation.

Together, the body of research looking at the relationship between emotion and cognition reveals that in many cases, signals of emotion are processed by the brain automatically and that this early detection of emotion can influence a range of cognitive functions, including perception, attention, memory, and decision making. Conversely, a range of cognitive functions can affect the experience of emotion (Phelps 2006). Following on the work of Damasio (1994) and others, Leung, Epstein, and Moulton (Chapter 7) writing on cognition and competence within the health professions, suggest, "The historical separation of thinking and feeling has largely been replaced by the prevailing view that cognition and emotion processes are integral to each other and operate in parallel." While we have gained significant knowledge regarding the interchange of emotion and cognition, there is still significantly more to learn and an impressive amount of research is being conducted along these lines.

In the health professions, these concepts have not been well integrated into our understanding of competency. Attempts at understanding motor skill acquisition, clinical-reasoning and decision-making skills, transfer of knowledge, and team performance are very much grounded in a purely cognitive approach, with virtually no discussion of the role of feelings and moods on these processes.

However, there is a growing interest in this area, with medical educators and researchers now designing studies to examine how cognitive reframing may help students reduce their anxiety when approaching difficult clinical tasks (De Souza and Solomon 2009). Another development in this area has been the study of the effects of anxiety on performance by residents during objective structured clinical exams (OSCE) (LeBlanc et al. 2008) and objective structured assessment of technical skills (OSATS) (LeBlanc and Bandiera 2007).

Our ideas about emotion influence our questions about it and, in turn, our research methods and what we count as evidence, all of which have repercussions for the kinds of knowledge claims we can make. For example, the idea that emotion can be measured through biological proxy measures such as changes in heart rate, cortisol levels in saliva, or skin conduction tests is inductive and directs us to look for evidence of emotion through observable mechanisms such as decision making and feats of memory. This approach differs from a neuroscientific one in which scientists directly access the physical changes in brain chemistry and structure, arriving at different findings, such as neurochemical imbalances, and different solutions. Emotions seen as effects of social and cultural factors produce methods and analysis of another kind. A social science perspective suggests that although we all experience joy, sadness, and anger, we do so in different ways for different reasons and, as much as they are recognized as internal and universal, emotions also make us unique through the ways in which they are connected to our social world. Emotion therefore can be examined as a psychological phenomenon, a neurophysiological process, and a sociocultural practice.

A Sociocultural Perspective

The cognitive and neurosciences contribute to our knowledge of the workings of perception, memory, and decision making, with important findings for fields such as education in understanding the role of emotion in performance and learning. The extent of this contribution, however, can be greatly enhanced with improved understanding of the social environments in which learning and clinical performance take place (Bruer 1997). Such a perspective moves from a view interior to the individual to one that looks at emotion and our understanding of emotion as shaped by the social world.

From a sociocultural viewpoint, emotions are seen as collaboratively constructed and distributed among individuals in particular cultural and social contexts and are studied for their effect in the world rather than for their composition. By focusing on emotions not as biologically or privately experienced phenomena but rather as part of shifting social performances, we can recognize that they are "productive of experiences and constitutive of realities...and the truths with which we work" (Lutz and Abu-Lughod 1990, 10). In the field of cognition the concept of attunement and collaborative cognition are brought to mind. In the context of health care teams, "attunement and collaborative cognition among members of a team or an organization can contribute to sense making in which collective brainstorming and sharing experiences generate meaning" (Leung, Epstein, and Moulton, Chapter 7).

Such a perspective directs our attention to emotion's function in social exchanges and its role as social, political, and cultural mediator. Social science approaches then foreground emotion as a practice rather than a neurochemical process. Emotion becomes visible in this realm as skills, a component of our character, and as a form of labor. In the following sections we will explore these different, socially derived constructions of emotion and their implications for competency.

Emotional Intelligence and Emotional Regulation

As reviewed in the sections above, emotions are integral to a person's ability to process, interpret, remember information, and make decisions about the world around him/her. Additionally, they shape and can be shaped by social, cultural, and political forces. In recognition of the role of emotion in individual, social, cultural, and political life, some systematic approaches toward the development or training of emotional management as a skill have emerged, notably emotional intelligence and emotional regulation.

Emotional Intelligence

Emotional intelligence (EI) is the most prevalent explanatory framework for understanding emotion within the business, leadership, and organization professions today, as well as within health professional training. This model sits on the border between psychological and sociological attempts to explain emotions as powerful mediators in the social world. EI meets health care's humanistic goals of developing caring professionals while providing a dependable method for measuring and judging capacities seen as not otherwise amenable to reliable capture. EI in health professional education frames emotions as skills to be honed through practice. Emotions are seen as mutable despite being also hardwired in our neurophysiology and are the sole responsibility of the individual to change for the better. EI makes it possible to observe and assess emotion as a skilled behavior.

The term *emotional intelligence* was popularized by Daniel Goleman in his 1995 best seller, *Emotional Intelligence: Why It Can Matter More Than IQ*. Despite much ongoing competition between different versions and interpretations of emotional intelligence as a concept, the most popular and well-known model is Goleman's. His model of EI combines skills, abilities, and personality traits. It rationalizes different emotional competencies such as emotional management, along quasi-neuroscientific lines. Emotional management, for instance, involves the amygdala or other "emotion centers" (Goleman 1995, 19). Goleman bases his claims on the neuroscientific discoveries of Joseph LeDoux (1996) and Antonio Damasio (1994). He clusters competencies related to emotional intelligence under four domains: self-awareness, self-management, social awareness, and relationship management. Each domain is described with accompanying abilities. For example, the self-management domain includes the competency of trustworthiness, and individuals who demonstrate this competency are authentic and reliable.

Searching the terms "emotional intelligence" and "medical education" will bring up well over one thousand books and over two hundred thousand articles, suggesting that there is a full-scale uptake of this discourse within medical education specifically as it relates to competence as a practice of skills. In "Becoming an Emotionally Intelligent Physician," Mitchell Feldman suggests that "the core competencies involved in emotional intelligence are the perception of emotions (in self and others), the understanding of these emotions, and the management of emotions." He goes on to say this understanding is a "prerequisite to achieving personal growth, essential in the skilled management of emotions in medical practice (such as the use of empathy)" (2001, 98). In another article, "Emotion Skills Training for Medical Students," Satterfield and Hughes (2007) review emotional skills education programs using the same language as Feldman and focusing on "the category of emotion skills or the teachable set of cognitive and behavioral strategies that facilitate emotional awareness, understanding and management" (941).

Thinking about emotion as an individual's skill set resonates with the cognitive behavioral notion of emotion as alterable. That is, our emotions can be changed through individual training and practice. It also dovetails with the blossoming simulation technologies that suggest, like EI, that emotion can be improved through inter- and intrapersonal communication skills coaching.

EI models are currently applied to everything from medical school admissions processes (Carrothers, Gregory, and Gallagher 2000) to studies looking at the possible relationship between EI attributes and students' clinical skills as assessed by standardized patients (Elam, Stratton, and Andrykowski 2001). Critical voices urge caution against a naive and full-scale uptake of EI, suggesting that "there is a lack of conceptual clarity surrounding the whole notion of EI, with different models and measures, contradictory reliability and validity studies of the measurement tools and little critical analysis (at least in the medical education literature)" (Lewis et al. 2005, 340).

Emotional Regulation

Related to the concept of emotional intelligence is the concept of emotional regulation: the cognitive regulation of emotional responses and states as a complement to normal social function and adaptive interactions with the environment. Through conscious strategies and practice, it is thought that individuals can change their interpretation of specific emotional stimuli, and thus can alter their emotional reactions (Phelps 2006). This was demonstrated by Ochsner and colleagues (2002), who asked study participants to look at pictures of emotional scenes, such as a picture of women crying outside a church. One group of participants was asked to simply pay attention to their natural emotional reactions. Another group was asked to reappraise the situation, so that rather than interpreting the image as women crying in grief at the funeral of a loved one, they were to interpret the image as women crying in joy at a wedding. These reappraisals were able to alter the experience of emotion and to diminish activation of the amygdala, suggesting that reappraisals can lead to modifications in the emotional responses.

A practical application of emotional regulation is stress inoculation training (Meichenbaum 1996). The objective of the training is to prepare individuals to respond more favorably to stressful events and to depathologize stress reactions. The first phase of the training is the conceptual/education phase, in which the goal is to help individuals gain a better understanding of the nature of stress and its effects. Next is the skill acquisition and rehearsal phase. The aim of this phase is the development and practice of coping skills to reduce anxiety and enhance the individual's capacity to respond effectively to stressful situations. This phase is focused on training the individual to maintain an awareness of stress reactions and to invoke appropriate skills to reduce stress. These skills consist of cognitive restructuring techniques aimed at regulating negative emotions and thoughts, and relaxation techniques to increase control over physiological responses. The third and final step is the application phase. The coping skills are applied in increasingly stressful conditions that approximate the real-world stressor environment. Stress inoculation training has been found to be effective in reducing general state anxiety and performance anxiety (anxiety specific to the skills being addressed in the training) and in enhancing performance under stress (Driskell, Johnston, and Salas 2001; Gaab et al. 2003, 2006; Hammerfald, Eberle, and Grau 2006; Johnston and Cannon-Bowers 1996; Saunders et al. 1996).

Expressions of emotion are important aspects of health professional training and performances of competence. Demonstration of emotion regulation is central to professional concepts such as "detached concern" as a sign of competency. In medicine, learning to manage one's emotional expression is carried out through practice, which is elevated in importance through performance assessment activities. Research suggests that cognitive and social functions can be changed in emotional settings, so training that focuses solely on cognitive aspects is unlikely to adequately prepare individuals to function in highly emotional crisis situations. The literature reviewed in this chapter suggests that the concept of emotional regulation is worthy of further inquiry and exploration. This needs to be done carefully, however, and by examining the consequences of this training. While approaches to regulating emotions do lead to immediate reductions in subjective and physiological responses, suppression of emotions has the opposite effect, along with less desired social consequences (Glass and McKnight 1996). Furthermore, the long-term mental and physical effects of emotional suppression are not fully understood.

Emotion in a cognitive behavioral discourse such as EI is seen a skill or tool that can be honed through practice; it is observable as a demonstrable behavior. Ideas about emotional competency are supported by educational approaches such as EI that rely on the visibility of emotion to make judgments about professionalism.

Emotion and Competency: "To Do" or "To Be"

As we have discussed, social science perspectives convey the idea of emotions as part of a tool kit of skills as supported by an emotional intelligence and an emotional regulation framework, but the medical education literature also constructs emotions as a marker of character formation. The first perspective supports a particularly instrumental and regulatory adoption of emotion to which individual practitioners are subjected through practice and assessment, while the second sees emotion as a commodity. A character formation perspective describes emotion and its management as a component of an individual's values, attitudes, and beliefs. Internalized attributes and characteristics defined according to professional ideals are nurtured and abstracted into competencies. The idea of competency as a set of skills focuses on "doing the right thing," while the idea of emotion as a unique aspect of one's character focuses on remediating the internal moral ethical landscape of the individual, or "being the right thing."

"Doing the Right Thing"

Within a framework that constructs emotion as a practice, competency is made visible through demonstrations of communication skills while also being linked to empathy as a particular type of performance. For example, medical trainees observed in acts of demonstrating competency in the skill of suturing can be assessed for both the performance of technique and success of outcome. The same rationale exists for demonstrating emotion as a skill. To demonstrate is to focus on the activity of "doing to," which is observable as an outcome. In the case of emotion as a communication skill, the outcome is the effect of the competent encounter (calmer, more compliant patient or colleague). Empathy becomes a technique—"the how" of the skill carried out. There are a number of heuristic tools for reminding learners about how to express empathy, such as Robert Buckman's "S-P-I-K-E-S" model for delivering bad news, which lays out specific steps one can take to achieve empathic competence and provides an acronym by which to remember them (Buckman 2005). Practicing empathy as part of a communication skill—as commonly done with standardized patients, for example—has the potential to turn it into a rehearsal or practice of a manipulation. Hanna and Fins (2006), writing about the effect of altered power relations in simulated patient teaching, suggest that

> a medical student may, through practice in simulation encounters, be able to
> master all the skills and tricks of surface communication and be able to use

them very effectively in an OSCE and in later practice effectively.... [But] does he or she ever learn to master the discursive and ontological power that makes the physician-patient relationship an invigorated, productive lived reality rather than a set of acting techniques? (267)

An outcomes approach that suggests human connection can be learned and assessed as a demonstration of technique may be creating new realities where the performed comes to stand in for the "real" and define it in new ways. Such possibilities are supported by performance examinations like objective structured clinical examinations (OSCEs) in which there is pressure both to dissimulate—or to "not act"—that which is present (e.g., disdain, anger) as well as to simulate—performing "as if" one cared— according to standardized checklists. As one student reported, "The only time that I feel like [I am] faking is when [I] try to be empathic. It is odd, I think, to express empathy to somebody when you know they don't really have the condition" (Hodges 2007, 127).

Judgments about the acceptability of emotional skills are made possible by technologies that support systems of observation. Psychometrics, highly formalized performance/demonstration protocols, observation guides and performance checklists, assessment and feedback, video and digital technology, and standardized patients (SPs) are given legitimacy. The ways in which one participates in this assemblage includes SPs as teachers, acting coaches, and in some cases assessors; students as performers; and clinicians as expert observers. All are legitimized and given roles by constructing the invisible as something that needs to be regulated as a skill.

Constructing emotion and social processes as skills that can be learned, practiced, improved, and evaluated makes alignment with a professional norm possible. It also justifies comparison between individuals about their emotional competency as it relates to professional notions of appropriate behavior. However, viewing emotion as simply another set of skills in our cognitive tool kit, although practical, does not go far enough in recognizing the need to move beyond explanatory models that put all the responsibility for managing, controlling, and explaining emotion on the individual. While it is helpful to have ways of practicing skills related to emotional behavior, health professionals, trainees, and patients are not well served by these alone.

"Being the Right Thing"

An equally pervasive and long-standing framework for understanding emotion as a component of competence within the health professions constructs it as an essential part of practitioner professional identity. Our attention is directed to an individual's internal moral character, values, attitudes, and beliefs. Professionalism as a process of identity formation is interested both in how professionalism is internalized and in the socio-historical forces that structure and regulate normative definitions—or how to become a doctor and a member of the medical profession (Brosnan and Turner 2009, 70). An identity formation view of emotion focuses on a health professional's capacity for empathy over the practical aspects of how to communicate it; or as one educator put it: "How can we stop the rot?" (Spencer 2004). Empathy can be seen as the most privileged and visible site of medicine's concern regarding the status of emotion in the profession and its moral failure to produce "good" humanistic doctors. The process of training related to identity has been named "professional formation" by its authors, with the stated "goal of anchor[ing] students to foundational principles while helping them navigate the inevitable moral conflicts of medicine" (Rabow et al. 2010, 310).

Increasing emphasis placed on self-reflection as a necessary competency is part of an educational technology that posits emotion not as a skill but as "a mechanism that can be used to internalize a professional ethos of self-regulation" (Hodges 2006, 694). Emotion, together with cognition, is the main object and mechanism of self-reflection: How does one feel about "the encounter," "the decision," "what just happened"? Self-reflection can become part of the moral architecture for developing physicians: "Through written discussion of critical incidents and professionalism evaluations, students can *demonstrate* their ability for self-reflection, discernment of relevant values, and actions they have taken based on their values" (Rabow et al. 2010, 315; emphasis added). Successful "professional formation" is apparent through alignment of an individual's self-reflections with the values and attributes put forward by the dominant professionalism discourse. In other words, professionalism is the successful outcome of the competent internalization of normative moral values.

In an article entitled "Professional Formation: Extending Medicine's Lineage of Service into the Next Century" (Rabow et al. 2010), the authors suggest that "when individual physicians cannot be counted on to act with personal integrity, not only is the doctor–patient relationship threatened but the social contract with the profession of medicine is fractured as well" (312). Emotions are described as instruments of moral persuasion that "ensure physicians are prepared to lead lives of compassion and service" (ibid., 310). In this framing of professional competency, emotion emerges as a kind of morality and ethics. Its focus is on the professional's integrity of character and fashions medicine as a "calling," reflecting the connection between medicine and religion and positioning medical work as sacred and sacrificial.

In an approach that frames emotion as essentially moral, medical training that focuses on evidence-based approaches, problem-based learning, and performance assessments is seen by some to degrade the humane aspects of professional practice (Rabow et al. 2010). Rather, professional socialization processes are meant to instill proper values, such as commitment to community service, converting students to a sense of stewardship and social responsibility in the process. Increased "values training" is validated through writing on the decline of empathy in medical students, which focuses on it as a characteristic of the individual. Competencies related to self-reflection, self-assessment, mindfulness, and inclusion of the humanities, which on their own may offer critical space for community and identity formation, may be co-opted by a regulatory agenda that asks students to reflect in the "right" way on the "right" moral material in order to produce the "good" health professional. In this way, emotion as a competency becomes embedded in professional morality and through training experiences becomes internalized as commonsense truths (Boler 1999, 39).

Emotion as Labor

Another contribution to the study of emotion in the professional world examines it as a form of labor. A shift has occurred, according to Miller (2007), both as a result of a move away from the moral models mentioned above and as part of a global economic progression from manufacturing to human service occupations. She suggests that "organizational participants are coping with new challenges, and those challenges often involve complex processes of emotion in the workplace" (224). The literature on emotional labor concentrates on emotion as a commodity that is used for the sake of profit. Yet for many human service workers, like health care professionals, the emotion involved in the job is not manufactured for profit, but is a human part of both the work being done and the person doing the work (ibid.).

Pioneering work in the area has been carried out by sociologist Arlie Hochschild, who studied emotion in service occupations, such as the restaurant and airline fields, examining the gendered nature of emotion as work (2003). In *The Managed Heart* (2003), she defines emotional labor as an activity that "requires one to induce or suppress feeling in order to sustain the outward countenance that produces the proper state of mind in others" (7). The criteria she uses to define emotional labor includes face-to-face interaction, handling of other people's feelings and one's own, and the expression of emotion, such as smiling, as part of a job description (11). In health professional work, as in any work requiring human contact, there are implicit "feeling rules" requiring certain behaviors to be performed or repressed for the good of the patient, the professional, and the profession itself. For example, the act of counseling patients about behavior that is dangerous to their health, such as smoking, presupposes a caring relationship as a motivating element in the hoped-for behavior change. In fact, the patient's behavior may incite feelings of disgust or anger in the practitioner. Yet both the performance of compassionate emotion and the suppression of angry ones, along with a necessary attitude of support, is part of the physician's therapeutic emotional labor in this instance. Emotion is central to the work carried out by health care professionals daily. Understanding emotion, reflecting on emotion, engaging with emotion, and expressing emotion are important work-related aspects of competent practice.

A broad range of ideas and theories has been covered in our examination of emotion as a form of health professional competency. Not all of them are in agreement with each other. As mentioned at the beginning of the chapter though, it is our contention that each of the views and accompanying theories contributes to a greater understanding of the role of emotion in professional training and practice. Our contention is that a naive and undertheorized understanding of emotion in the health professions acts as a barrier to appreciating more fully the contributions different views offer us. In the following sections, we summarize some of the implications that compartmentalized or naive thinking about emotion produces and offer suggestions for a more comprehensive integration of emotion into health professional training in the future.

Implications of the Current Ideas about Emotion within the Health Professions

Although most health professionals would agree that emotions are a regular element of clinical practice, that they shape behavior and thoughts, and that they are worthy of discussion, a closer look suggests that we tend to view them as illegitimate and undesired, devalue them in relation to reason, and ignore them in designing health professional curricula. We suggest that a shift in the way in which emotions are conceived of in the health professions is overdue for the following reasons.

Despite the increasing recognition over the last two decades of emotion as "socially constructed," the view of emotion as individualized and gendered is deeply embedded in our language and conceptual frameworks and is realized in a skills-based approach to emotional competency. Implications of this suggest that increased student and practitioner isolation and burnout are individualized and private. Emotions identified as outside the norm of acceptable can remain hidden, to be handled individually by "getting control of yourself" or "putting feelings aside." A skill-based view of emotion maintains a conception of learning as an individual endeavor. Emotions are constructed as static and simple, available to be measured along a continuum of functioning and skill, rather than as complex and part of a dynamic cultural process.

With the exception of work now being undertaken by a few researchers such as Moulton and colleagues (2007, 2010a, 2010b), emotions are largely ignored both in scientific endeavors to understand how competency and experience are acquired and in educational and professional socialization processes. For example, the study of clinical reasoning and decision making, although including elements of unconscious automatic processes, has focused on purely cognitive elements. In teaching interpersonal and communication skills, we use rubrics that reflect cognitive aspects of diagnostics and management as reasoning processes, while emotion is present either as a demonstration of skills such as listening or as a marker of ability related to moral character. In dividing emotion from cognition in this way, we give value to reason as if it were separate from and more important than emotion. Given the important role that emotions play in our ability to process information and interact in social environments, our attempts to explain behavior, learning, and social interactions stand to gain in sophistication by incorporating emotional components.

By valuing reason and logic over emotions, we also run the risk of inadvertently promoting emotional suppression as desirable. In doing so, we may be creating situations and learning conditions that are favorable to the development of burnout and other negative long-term sequelae. Other risks exist in the uncritical adoption of the EI or emotional regulation technologies as an approach to professional competency (Lewis et al. 2005). Raising awareness of emotions, learning to manage one's own emotions, and using newly acquired knowledge to improve social success are not problems in themselves. Who of us doesn't see the benefit of being more emotionally aware and of developing skills to navigate social and professional situations more successfully? However, the naive uptake of complex neuroscientific processes and the simplistic application and rationalization of quasi-scientific methods diminish the growing sophistication in the area of emotion studies. In fact, "the construct of emotion itself is extremely complex and still poorly understood and research in this field is still developing" (Lewis et al. 2005, 349).

Furthermore, by lacking a clear understanding of the role of emotion in the cognitive and social worlds of individuals, we run the risk of adopting unformulated strategies in attempting to integrate emotions into our conceptions of competency. An educator who believes that trainees learn better under pressure without fully understanding the complex interactions between emotions and memory runs the risk of creating learning situations where the source of emotions is separate from the information that is to be learned. An obvious example is the case of an educator who teaches by intimidation or shame in an attempt to make the students remember the information better. In such a case, the students are more likely to remember the teacher rather than the information presented.

Finally, incomplete understanding of the relationship of emotion with competency can lead to an overly simplistic incorporation of emotion in ways that are internally inconsistent. For example, students are selected into medical school partly on the basis of demonstrated behaviors that reveal a high degree of empathy (Parry et al. 2006), yet we systematically erode these characteristics by repeatedly placing them in highly emotional situations without addressing the impact that this has, and we value suppression of emotions in favor of reason and logic.

The Way Forward: Integrating Emotions into our Conceptualization of Competency

Recognizing emotion as a form of knowledge production that is as valuable as rationality in professional and personal functioning would entail a number of collaborative moves on the part of scientists who hold different views about emotion. Coming to the understanding that many of our ideas overlap may offer opportunities for extending understanding about the role of emotion as a competency and contribute to each others' work in important ways.

There will always be tension between approaches that view emotion as a neurological, cognitive, or sociocultural phenomenon. Yet this should not stop us, as researchers and educators, from addressing emotion as an essential form of epistemology and acknowledging its importance with respect to health professional competence. Health professionals, health professional trainees, and patients/clients are negatively affected by the current tendency to pathologize or omit emotion from current thinking about competence. We need to collectively acknowledge and work with emotions in ways that honor them as internal and individual, as well as socially and culturally constructed, while also questioning the split between emotion and rationality.

Suggestions for integrating emotion into the health professions as a form of competency include designing research programs in which different aspects of emotion are examined with respect to issues of competency. Using the example of reasoning, one could look at how reasoning changes in various emotional situations, such as the role of regret or stress on clinical reasoning and decision making. Creating educational and research forums in which different ideas about emotion in health professional practice are discussed (not assessed) could offer opportunities for producing new understanding and acceptance of emotion in professional practice. Writing emotion explicitly into curriculum, especially as it relates to clinical decision making and problem solving, would improve our awareness of the role of emotion in day-to-day practice. Despite the emotional nature of clinical training and practice, there is little direct reference to emotion in formal educational and professional documents. Also, as mentioned throughout this chapter, challenging naive and unformulated integration of emotions into practice is important. At best, the resulting knowledge from naive or unformulated integration of emotions will be ineffective. At worst, perpetuating the dichotomy between emotion and reason will be detrimental to students, practicing health professionals, and the profession itself. Social, cultural, and political beliefs about emotion are powerful forces for producing and reproducing notions of professional competence with implications for practice and the health professions. Emotion as a form of competence, we contend, needs to be recognized for its central role in health professional training.

4

Competence as Expertise

Exploring Constructions of Knowledge in Expert Practice

Maria Mylopoulos

Excellence in the education and training of future experts is crucial to the success of all professions. Extensive efforts have therefore been made to explore expertise, with the aim of translating understanding of expert performance into more effective expert development. However, our understanding of what it means to perform at the highest levels of a profession and the particular competencies that we value as the core of excellence have proven to be dynamic, and often controversial, issues. Over the last half century, the accrual and organization of an extensive knowledge base have become widely accepted by educators and researchers as the foundation for expertise and expert performance. The dominance of the view of acquired knowledge as the foundation for expertise is mirrored in the many competency frameworks that foreground the application of clinical knowledge, skills, and procedures, even as they seek to be inclusive of additional competencies. Meanwhile, as our understanding of expertise has expanded to include previously unexplored facets of expert performance, the particular role of knowledge in expert development and practice is being increasingly revisited. In particular, the ability of practitioners not only to apply their knowledge to routine problems but also to deal with novel, emergent, or unexpected problems of practice effectively, and to use these experiences as the basis for a process of continual improvement, is not adequately accounted for by models of expertise that conceptualize problem solving as the application of acquired knowledge.

In this chapter I will explore various cognitive constructions of expertise, with a particular focus on the differing ways in which the role of accrued knowledge has been conceptualized in models of expert development and practice. I will discuss key implications for those seeking to understand competence through the lens of expert performance. First, "knowledge in the head" will be explored, including conceptualizations of knowledge as they relate to the individual practitioner and the implications for understanding learning. The second section will be an elaboration of the constructions and implications of moving knowledge beyond the individual and into "the world," including knowledge embedded in communities and contexts. Finally, implications for notions of competence in health professions education will be discussed.

Knowledge in the Head

Traditional models of expertise have focused on experts' ability to apply knowledge effectively and efficiently to recurring problems of practice. Research across domains of performance has explored expert-novice differences to investigate the question of what an expert has "in the head." These bodies of knowledge have highlighted the importance of the acquisition and organization of knowledge, as well the vital role of practice in acquiring the necessary knowledge to build expertise. Knowledge in this framework is thus understood as a resource, making it possible for experts to apply their extensive knowledge base to problems of practice.

The Answer-Filled Practitioner

Arguably, the current dominant view of expertise, both from a lay and research perspective, is the construction of the expert as the "go to" person who has the answers to the most challenging problems in their domain

(Norman 2005b). This perspective is grounded in an extensive body of research comparing expert and novice problem solving that has identified differences in knowledge structures accounting for much of the efficiency, automaticity, and depth of understanding integral to expert problem solving—and absent in novice problem solving (Elstein, Shulman, and Sprafka 1978). It has been argued that these novice/expert differences demonstrate the primacy of knowledge, and more specifically the importance of how knowledge is organized in the expert's head, in the process of expert problem solving. For example, a brief look at the clinical reasoning literature highlights the variety of strategies, cognitive structures, and mechanisms that experts rely on in their problem solving. Researchers have argued that the expert knowledge base is organized through knowledge encapsulations (van de Wiel, Boshuizen, and Schmidt 2000), illness scripts (Charlin et al. 2007), and semantic axes (Bordage and Lemieux 1991). Medical experts have been shown to make use of instances (Norman and Brooks 1997), mathematical probabilities, and pattern recognition (Elstein et al. 2000) to arrive at a diagnosis. This range of mechanisms, structures, and processes that characterizes expert clinical reasoning suggests that experts do not just have more knowledge than novices, but rather that the organization and coordination of different types of knowledge is vital to expert performance (Eva 2005).

The centrality of knowledge acquisition in this framework of expertise leads to a conceptualization of expert development as a journey along which knowledge and experience are acquired (Schmidt and Boshuizen 1993). In order to become an expert, one needs to acquire extensive amounts of domain-specific knowledge and experience, and through this prolonged, guided process of acquisition, one gradually develops the knowledge structures best suited to expert problem solving (Custers, Regehr, and Norman 1996; Ericsson, Krampe, and Teschromer 1993). For example, a developing physician on the path from novice to expert will be expected to gain various types of knowledge, including basic science mechanisms, clinical signs and symptoms, case examples, and technical skills. At first, the mental representation of this knowledge will include organized facts and a limited set of heuristics and reasoning strategies. Over time, however, through classroom instruction and hands-on experience with a variety of cases, the developing expert clinician will gradually acquire greater amounts of knowledge and begin to organize and access this information in a manner that may be fundamentally different from the novice (Schmidt and Boshuizen 1993). Importantly, the novice/expert comparisons that dominate this literature suggest that expertise is the inevitable result of a developmental pathway consisting of appropriate training and sufficient amount of practice (Mylopoulos and Regehr 2007).

While the literature exploring the precise organization of knowledge and its impact on expert problem solving is abundant and continues to evolve, other facets of expert performance are increasingly shifting attention away from the construction of the expert solely as an "answer-filled" practitioner.

Knowledge as Efficiency: "Freeing Up"
Resources for Further Cognitive Activity

While experts are unquestionably able to solve problems more effectively than novices, other explorations of expert/expert differences have led researchers to consider dimensions of expert practice that extend beyond the ability to apply knowledge to solve problems (Bransford, Brown, and Cocking 2000; Hatano and Inagaki 1986; Schwartz, Bransford, and Sears 2005). Specifically, the ability of experts to use problem solving as an opportunity to learn, construct new knowledge, and engage in sustained practice improvement has increasingly been framed as a core competency of "true expert" performance (Bereiter and Scardamalia 1993). In this conceptualization, an extensive, structured knowledge base remains central and necessary for expertise. However, rather than conceptualizing expert problem solving solely as the application of knowledge, the exploration and inclusion of these additional facets of expert performance has elaborated the role that knowledge plays in expertise.

Research exploring distinctions between experts is grounded in the impact that knowledge has on expertise beyond problem solving per se. For example, Bereiter and Scardamalia (1993) argue that "true experts" engage in a process of "progressive problem-solving," using the knowledge they acquire to routinize certain aspects of their practice, thereby allowing them to invest more cognitive resources into constructing and addressing increasingly complex representations of problems of practice. Knowledge in this conceptualization has a dual role: both to provide answers to problems that are well-known and to enable the use of additional cognitive resources for continuing excellence in practice. In contrast, "experienced nonexperts" are understood to be content to use their extensive knowledge base to solve problems without an accompanying reinvestment of cognitive resources. Crucially, in this model, true experts can become experienced nonexperts if they do not maintain their commitment to sustained practice improvement, which is characterized as working to improve even while practicing at the highest levels of performance in their domain.

Parallel research programs have elaborated the construct of adaptive expertise. Similar to the true experts, articulated by Bereiter and Scardamalia, adaptive experts work within what has been termed the "optimal adaptability corridor," balancing complementary efficiency and innovation dimensions of practice. This balancing allows adaptive experts to use knowledge to solve problems efficiently and effectively (like experienced nonexperts) and to create new knowledge when facing novel problems of practice (Schwartz, Bransford, and Sears 2005). The complementary nature of these two dimensions of expertise cannot be overstated; the crux of effective adaptive expert practice is the effective balance between using existing knowledge and constructing new knowledge in response to problems of practice. In this way, performance is maintained and also continuously improved. Crucial to adaptive expert practice is the assumptive nature of knowledge; that is, the view of experts not as answer-filled but rather as "accomplished novices" who use their deep understanding of the knowledge within their domain to challenge the status quo and consistently push the boundaries of what is known (Bransford, Brown, and Cocking 2000).

The recognition of differences in performance between experts has brought to the fore the reality that not every individual who completes the recognized trajectory of expert development achieves excellence in their chosen domain (Hatano and Inagaki 1986). In spite of our assessment of ourselves as above average (see Eva, Regehr, and Gruppen in chapter 6 of this volume), most individuals merely "swell the ranks of the mediocre" (Bereiter and Scardamalia 1993). While the knowledge-based trajectory culminating in the "answer-filled expert" has been conceptualized as a spontaneous trajectory of development, researchers exploring adaptive expertise argue that there are two "spontaneous" trajectories of expertise, one leading to adaptive expertise, or the development of a "true expert," and the other leading to routine expertise, or the development of an "experienced nonexpert" (Hatano and Inagaki 1986). The key to developing adaptive expertise is maintaining the balance between efficiency and innovation throughout development. Developing experts should not solely focus on acquiring an extensive knowledge base for problem solving, but should also develop their ability to construct knowledge in response to novel problems; they should adopt a stance toward knowledge that will enable them to view their knowledge base as assumptive, falsifiable, improvable, and dynamic rather than a static database for problem solving. In order to do so, trainees must be provided with opportunities to exercise both dimensions of expert practice throughout their development (Schwartz, Bransford, and Sears 2005).

Exploring the shifting role of knowledge across constructions of expertise has the potential to expand understanding of the ways in which knowledge underpins expert competencies. Knowledge maintains its role as a resource for problem solving, but there is a vital shift: knowledge now has a dual role, both as a resource for problem solving and also as a resource for knowledge creation and practice improvement. This expanded role of knowledge captures additional competencies of expertise—namely, the ability of experts to learn and improve their practice, and also to work at the boundaries of their domain, contributing new knowledge and understanding. While the two constructions of expertise elaborated thus far are representative of different literatures, there are crucial intersections that emphasize the complementary nature of these frameworks (Mylopoulos and Woods 2009). For example, while the necessity and importance of the efficiency dimension of practice has been well articulated in adaptive expertise research, it is nonetheless characterized as the "replicative and applicative" use of knowledge (Schwartz, Bransford, and Sears 2005). However, research on clinical reasoning has shown that the applicative and replicative uses of knowledge are complex phenomena. Therefore understanding the efficiency dimension of adaptive expertise through the lens of the "answer-filled expert" could have significant implications for our conceptualization of expert practice. For educators and researchers interested in evolving a fuller construct of expertise that incorporates both the "answer-filled" and "adaptive" constructions of expert, research exploring this more integrated construct of expertise could potentially have a significant impact toward articulating a more comprehensive set of competencies that form the foundation of expert practice.

Implications of the Role of Knowledge
for Transfer of Learning

The implications of the changing role of knowledge in constructions of expertise can be seen in resulting approaches to the phenomenon of transfer of learning. In particular, when the role of knowledge in expertise is understood as a database for problem solving and the primary competence of experts is to solve problems effectively and efficiently, the focus on "direct transfer" of knowledge from one problem to another is logical. However, shifting to a more elaborated role of knowledge and additional expert competencies necessarily changes the focus of what it means to transfer learning effectively.

Direct transfer of learning has been traditionally defined as the transfer of acquired knowledge from one problem-solving situation to another in order to solve a new problem; the concept is vital to the development and practice of expertise. Understanding and enhancing transfer of learning is therefore central to the efforts of educators and has been the focus of research since the beginning of the twentieth century (see Thorndike and Woodworth 1901). Over the course of this long history of research, researchers have typically used "sequestered problem solving" (SPS) methodology, where a learning session is followed by an SPS assessment requiring unassisted, direct application of previous learning (Bransford and Schwartz 1999). Using the SPS methodology, researchers have consistently found that transfer of learning is very difficult for learners; they typically display a 10–30 percent success rate in solving novel problems by applying appropriate solutions from previously solved problems (Norman 2009). For example, in one classic transfer problem, individuals learn an effective way of beaming X-rays at a tumor and then are asked to solve the problem of how crusaders can best attack a castle. When not prompted, learners are successful at transferring the solution for the tumor problem to the castle problem about 20 percent of the time. However, if learners are told that the solution for the first problem should lead to a solution for the second, 75 percent of them effectively transfer the solution across problems (Gick and Holyoak 1980). Essentially, transfer of learning is not automatic; individuals have to be looking for a relationship. Moreover, in order to solve analogous problems, learners must move beyond potentially misleading surface similarities and identify similarity at the deep, conceptual level of a problem. Research has shown that learners often tend to miss deep structure similarities and are easily misled by surface structure similarities and differences.

In contrast, the empirical story is different for individuals identified as experts (within the framework of the current discussion, these would be "answer-filled" experts), who tend to be better at transfer than novices due to their "domain enriched problem representation" (Norman 2009). For example, Chi, Feltovich, and Glase (1981) showed that expert physicists describe a particular problem as a "conservation of energy" problem, while novices refer to the same problem as a "ball rolling down a plane" problem, revealing the differences in the way experts and novices use their past knowledge to "see" new problems and lending credence to the importance of knowledge acquisition and organization in expert performance.

When moving to a view of knowledge as a resource for constructing new knowledge and expanding practice (rather than an exclusive interest in individuals' ability to apply knowledge from one problem-solving context to another), learning transfer is conceptualized as "preparation for future learning" (PFL) (Bransford and Schwartz 1999). PFL is understood as the ability to learn new information from available resources, relate new learning to past experiences, and demonstrate innovation and flexibility in problem solving. From this perspective, the important transfer of learning test is not to evaluate how well acquired knowledge can be applied to another problem, but rather how well acquired knowledge can facilitate the future learning of new, related knowledge. In contrast to traditional SPS methodology, which evaluates direct application of previous learning, PFL studies utilize a double transfer design (Bransford and Schwartz 1999; Schwartz and Bransford 1998). The double transfer design first engages participants in an initial learning session, followed by an opportunity to learn new, related knowledge, and then administers a final transfer test of their learning of the new knowledge. In this way the methodology explores both the transfer that helps individuals learn (transfer from the initial learning session to the new learning opportunity) and the transfer where one applies that learning (the new learning opportunity to the final transfer test). What researchers have found is that, when comparing different methods of instruction in the initial learning session, no differences are revealed between instructional methods when a standard SPS methodology is used (excluding the new learning opportunity). However, when each group is given the new learning opportunity, significant differences in performance are evident in the final transfer test. For example, one series of experiments compared two forms of instruction: the first centered on reading and summarizing a series of experiments in a particular domain, and the second focused on active analysis of simplified sets of data from sets of contrasting experiments in the same domain. Students who received instruction focused on active analysis were significantly more prepared to take advantage of the new learning opportunity compared to students who were asked to read and summarize (Bransford and Schwartz 1999). These results indicate that certain methods of instruction are superior for preparing learners to learn new knowledge when problem solving (Bransford and Schwartz 1999; Schwartz and Bransford 1998).

A PFL perspective to transfer of learning takes on particular importance when facing the reality that even the finest problem-solving instruction is unlikely to prepare clinicians for every problem-solving situation they may come across in their practice. In fact, PFL has been proposed as a key standard of performance for adaptive expertise (Bransford and Schwartz 1999), in that it focuses on the ability to transfer key adaptive expert competencies across problem-solving situations. Therefore, instead of focusing exclusively on SPS instruction and assessment, education researchers have argued that it is important for instruction and assessment to also include a focus on PFL. The task for education researchers is to find ways to optimize instruction in order to best support this form of learning and problem solving and to create assessments that can make the PFL ability observable as it develops. A shift from direct transfer to the inclusion of PFL in the conceptualization of what it means to be a competent learner and problem solver has significant implications for our understanding of expertise, expert development, and the competencies that we seek to foster throughout instruction and practice.

Beyond Knowledge in the Head

As models of expertise and expert development have begun to include additional competencies of expert performance, the conceptualization of the role of knowledge in expert problem solving has shifted from an exclusive emphasis on the ability to apply knowledge to problems of practice to the use of knowledge as the basis for innovation and flexibility in problem solving. Thus far in the discussion, the exploration of the role of knowledge has been restricted to what the individual expert has acquired "in their head"; however, theorists have been increasingly exploring the role of knowledge as it exists "in the world" and the ways in which these forms of knowledge might both define and shape additional expert competencies.

Knowledge as an Artifact

One way in which knowledge has been conceptualized as "in the world" is as an artifact, to be refined, improved, and elaborated by a knowledge-building community (Bereiter 2002; Bereiter and Scardamalia 2003; Scardamalia and Bereiter 2003a). This view of knowledge has taken on particular significance as experts are increasingly being called on to be the drivers of large-scale practice improvements in their domain. The ways in which experts share the knowledge they have constructed in response to novel problems of practice with their broader community takes on a key role in understanding the move "beyond best practice" in a given domain. In contrast to the diffusion literature (Rogers 1995), which centers on the diffusion and adoption of knowledge within communities, knowledge-building theory and other theories within the same paradigm (Bereiter 2002; Bereiter and Scardamalia 2003; Engeström 2001; Nonaka 1994; Scardamalia and Bereiter 2003a) examine knowledge sharing beyond the adoption of an idea, focusing instead on knowledge sharing for the purpose of collective idea improvement (Paavola, Lipponen, and Hakkarainen 2004). For example, knowledge-building theory positions knowledge sharing as part of an iterative process of creating knowledge through practice, thereby adding another step to the cycle of practice improvement that begins with true experts engaging in progressive problem solving in their daily work (Scardamalia and Bereiter 2003a). In this way, knowledge gained by experts through practice-based learning is conceptualized as an "improvable idea" that can be shared within a knowledge-building community for the purpose of collective and collaborative reflection and improvement. This articulation of the relationship between individual adaptive expert practice and sustained practice improvement at the community level is crucial, not least because it explicitly values ideas developed by experts in the course of their daily work (Mylopoulos and Scardamalia 2008).

The development of the skills necessary to function as part of a knowledge-building community is unquestionably important for sustained innovation within a domain. In order to achieve this aim, researchers within the knowledge-building paradigm have aimed to develop what have been termed *knowledge-building environments* (Bereiter and Scardamalia 2003). Working on the premise that immersion is a powerful way to prepare students to learn new ideas, collaboratively produce new knowledge, and innovate in new domains of work, educators and researchers have worked together to design classroom environments where these skills are integral to student success.

A knowledge-building environment (KBE) is any environment (virtual or otherwise) that enhances collaborative efforts to create and continually improve ideas (Scardamalia and Bereiter 2003b). There are two key features of a successful KBE. First, in order to enable the use of knowledge as an artifact, a KBE situates ideas beyond the minds of their creators and preserves them so that they can be available for collaborative idea improvement. In this way, the value of ideas is compounded over time in that collective achievements exceed individual contributions. Second, the dialogue fostered in a KBE supports idea diversity, constructive criticism and analysis, the organization of ideas into larger wholes, and the identification of recognized gaps and shortcomings of ideas. This democratic dialogue is fostered through the use of scaffolds, developed on the premise that "forms of discourse become forms of thinking" (Pontecorvo 1993). Scaffolds give ideas defined roles in such processes as theory refinement (e.g., having students begin sentences with "I need to understand...") and constructive criticism (e.g., "This theory cannot explain..."). The use of scaffolds in a KBE is not mandated, but is opportunistic, intended to help students embed these forms of discourse in their everyday work with ideas (Scardamalia 2004).

The understanding of knowledge as an artifact independent of both individuals and the context within which they exist creates opportunity and space for individuals to engage in productive work with ideas at the community level. Another way in which knowledge exists beyond the expert's head is as a situated construct, deeply embedded in the environments in which experts work.

Situated Knowledge

Expertise is enacted in a world filled with tools, technologies, and people, and expert performance is significantly impacted by the context in which experts find themselves working. From a distributed cognition perspective, that impact is not simply a question of mitigating quality of performance, but rather concerns the interactions between the knowledge that the expert brings to the problem-solving situation and the knowledge that is embedded in the social and physical environment within which the expert works. Thus, the role of knowledge situated in context is introduced to our understanding of expertise, and the ways in which experts successfully navigate their context to maximize performance become an important, and relatively unexamined, competency of expert performance. The theoretical framework of distributed cognition offers a lens through which to explore this competency, by seeking to understand the ways in which cognition might shape and be shaped by the social and physical contexts within which it occurs (Hutchins 1995; Pea 1993). Thus, cognition is understood to occur not as an isolated activity in the expert's mind, but as an activity in relation to the environment.

A distributed approach does not deny the importance of the knowledge the expert brings to the situation, but additionally acknowledges the importance of examining the knowledge the situation brings to the interaction. In this framework, knowledge is co-constructed by the individual and the situation (Brown, Collins, and Duguid 1989), and it is the interaction between the two, usually in the form of an activity to be observed, that is of interest. For example, Lave (1988) studied people grocery shopping, describing how shoppers' goals and solutions to problems are co-constructed by their initial intentions and expectations, the physical presentation of products, and the available resources for calculating the relative value of various purchases. Experts shape, construct, and manage their problem solving by taking advantage of affordances and removing barriers in the environment. At the same time, through this interactive process, those very affordances and barriers are shaping, and making possible, expert problem-solving goals and solutions. A distributed approach to understanding expert performance emphasizes the importance of particular expert competencies associated with complex, dynamic practice environments. It demands that knowledge be considered, not only as a resource in the individual expert's head or as an artifact in the world to be manipulated by expert communities, but also as a resource embedded in the particular problem-solving contexts and activities of experts.

The inclusion of situated knowledge into our understanding of expertise also requires a complementary shift in the ways in which we understand expert development. Sociocultural learning theories describe expert development as a situated phenomenon, recognizing the ways in which learning is embedded in the environments within which future experts are trained. For example, Lave and Wenger (1991) describe learning as an increasing familiarity with the affordances and constraints of an activity and the gradual movement of the learner from the periphery to a more central role in the practice of a community. In most clinical training models, a significant portion of learning takes place in clinical settings; therefore, it has been argued that sociocultural learning theories may provide more appropriate models of clinical learning by more accurately reflecting the situated nature of learning in these contexts (Bleakley 2006; Mann 2011). Essentially, there is an opportunity to teach trainees the ways in which context enables and constrains their practice and the ways in which they can purposefully use their context to extend the boundaries of their practice. Too often, however, the impact of context is left implicit for learners. In order to optimize development, these relationships could be more explicitly articulated and enabled, with guided opportunities to explore them from the earliest stages of development.

Revisiting Transfer of Learning in the Context of Knowledge in the World

The inclusion of knowledge in the world shifts the focus of interest when considering the phenomenon of transfer of learning. Bereiter (1995) has argued that when considering transfer, it is the "ability to behave intelligently" or the "transfer of disposition" across contexts that should be the focus of efforts aimed at improving transfer of learning. For example, Bereiter (1995) describes a fifth-grade science class learning about gravitational pull. From a traditional direct transfer perspective, the focus of transfer would be the students' ability to recognize new problems where gravitational pull would provide the necessary solution. From a transfer of disposition perspective, the transfer would be the quest for deeper understanding being carried over into new situations. For example, transfer might involve the types of questions asked when exploring the problem, ensuring that gaps in knowledge are addressed and exploring inconsistencies. When considering a world full of knowledge artifacts, Bereiter argues that the ability to behave intelligently is what enables experts to work effectively with ideas, producing new knowledge iteratively and collaboratively. The emphasis, according to Bereiter, should not be solely on transfer of concepts (direct transfer) or even transfer of the ability for future learning, but rather the ability to work effectively with knowledge artifacts.

The transfer of disposition perspective contrasts sharply with the position that situated learning theorists take on transfer of learning. At first glance, situated learning seems to provide an explanation of the failure of transfer; the more individuals become attuned to the particular barriers and affordances of a problem situation, the less likely it is that they will be able to transfer that knowledge usefully to other situations. Moreover, they will be faced with the challenge of overcoming learning that is counterproductive in a new situation, a phenomenon known as "negative transfer." Despite these challenges, however, a situated model of transfer has been articulated by Greeno, Smith, and Moore (1993), who define transfer of situated learning as the transfer of understanding of the constraints or affordances that are similar or dissimilar across problem-solving situations. In this way, individuals can determine whether their previous learning can have an effect in the new situation. Unlike previous, nonsituated accounts of transfer, the constraints and affordances are not characteristics of either the environment or of the individual independently, but rather are a feature of the relationship between individuals and their environment (Bereiter 1997).

Summary and Implications for Health Care

Ideally, every profession would be populated solely by experts, individuals performing at the highest levels of their chosen domain. In order to achieve this aim, education researchers have sought to define models of expertise that best reflect excellence in practice and to use this understanding to optimize trajectories of expert development. However, it is becoming increasingly clear, over decades of research, that the core competencies that underpin expert practice are topics of considerable debate among education researchers, resulting in divergent and sometimes competing paradigms of research on expertise. Perhaps most notably, the particular role of knowledge in constructions of expert practice and development has been the focus of considerable and divergent research programs, with significant implications for understanding and fostering expert practice and development in the professions.

In health care, the undisputed importance of effective clinical reasoning in practice has given rise to the dominance of the "answer-filled practitioner" in our conceptualization of expert health care professionals. However, increasingly, the realities of the dynamic, complex health care workplace have underscored the need for practitioners to be flexible, innovative, and adaptive in their practice and thereby highlighted the importance of recognizing and fostering the complementary role of knowledge as the basis for both the use of additional cognitive resources to advance problem solving and the construction of new knowledge. Moreover, as sustained practice improvement within health care has become an increasingly pressing imperative, the importance of understanding and fostering the use of knowledge as an artifact in expert communities for the process of sustained innovation is being emphasized (Mylopoulos and Scardamalia 2008). Finally, recognition of the significant impact of context on expert problem solving and learning has led to a consideration of the ways in which knowledge is situated in the contexts within which experts learn and practice. The inclusion of context in the understanding of expertise has highlighted the importance of considering the ways in which experts navigate the interaction between themselves and their environment (and concurrently, their knowledge and the knowledge situated in their environment). This issue is also central to Lingard's discussion earlier in this volume of competence in the context of teamwork (chapter 2). As she asserts, there is an aspect of expertise that is collectively negotiated and enacted. Perhaps the most challenging task for education researchers is to begin to reconcile our understanding of the myriad competencies of expertise discussed in this chapter with an integrated construct of expert practice (Mylopoulos and Regehr 2011).

As we consider what it means to be competent in health care practice, it is important to rethink *why* we know: we acquire knowledge not solely for the purpose of having all the answers but also for the purpose of challenging what we think we know, constructing new knowledge, and pushing the limits of our own best practice. Moreover, the inclusion of additional, previously unrecognized forms of knowledge into our understanding of what we can know, including knowledge as a community artifact for improvement and knowledge situated in the environments within which we work, would add richness to our understanding of what it means to be a competent expert in health care practice.

5

Assessing Competence

Extending the Approaches to Reliability

Lambert W. T. Schuwirth and Cees P. M. van der Vleuten

Prelude

The planning committee of the new Suntree Medical School was meeting to design a new assessment program for the curriculum. The members of the committee quickly agreed that the program should be fair, transparent, and defensible. They also agreed to make it as comprehensive as possible, covering not only "hard" factual knowledge but also skills, insights, attitudes, and professional abilities. On top of that, they realized the importance of including both modular and longitudinal elements of assessment.

At this point the committee got stuck. How were they going to reconcile the notions of fairness, transparency, and defensibility with the multifaceted assessment program they had in mind? It was pretty obvious to the members that fairness, transparency, and defensibility were easily demonstrable for the "hard" factual parts of the assessment program. They knew that the psychometric discourse, with its notions of construct validity and reliability, offers an excellent approach to the assessment of factual knowledge. But solutions for the "softer" parts of the assessment program were not so readily available. How to determine the reliability of observations in clinical practice and of repeated observations over a longer training period? Doesn't the object of measurement, the student, change over time? And what about the risk of such changes being interpreted as errors in the longitudinal measurements?

At this point, one committee member complicated matters further still by proposing a programmatic approach to assessment, one that would sometimes entail combining assessment results across instruments instead of only within single instruments. While this proposal clearly had merits, it confronted committee members with some really hard questions. To take one example: How would they ever be able to *reliably* combine a clinical supervisor's qualitative feedback on an abdominal examination with results on the abdominal anatomy items from an internal medicine test? Yet for a programmatic approach such combinations made sense, considering evidence that assessment scores generalize better across similar content than across similar formats. Moreover, such combinations would be needed for the level of integration aspired to in most views of competency-based education and assessment. Another question was: How to make a fair and defensible decision about a student's progress? And, finally, how were they to make fair and defensible decisions about individual students independently of the results of their peers?

When the deliberations had reached this stage, a clinician member of the committee suggested they abandon the idea that fairness, defensibility, trustworthiness, and credibility of assessment must invariably be approached from the traditional psychometric point of view: different methods may warrant different viewpoints. "It is the same in medicine," she said. "If I want to know the hemoglobin level of a patient, I don't want the lab analyst's opinion, I want a number. This may be 'objective,' purely numerical, determined in a standardized way, and norm referenced. For a pathology report, on the other hand, I don't want a number, I want a qualitative report; it does not matter if it is 'subjective' because I value the pathologist's expertise and opinions, and I want it to be criterion referenced, because it does not have to be related to the findings for other patients. The lab and pathology information combined tell me something about the patient's health, the necessary therapeutic actions, any further diagnostics, and the prognosis. If we decide to set up programmatic assessment for educational purposes and not merely for selection, we might want to try and mimic this approach and be prepared to define credibility, trustworthiness, and fairness in a more flexible way than in terms of reliability only."

Introduction

Assessment in education is important, and the stakes can be very high for all those involved. The debate can be heated, opinions are strong, and views manifold. Yet all stakeholders agree that assessment must be fair and trustworthy, procedures and methods must be up to current standards, results must be credible, and the whole assessment process must be taken seriously. Two characteristics of assessment, "validity" and "reliability," play a central role in this. But while the concept of validity has been debated extensively and has changed and evolved over time (Kane 2006), the concept of reliability seems to have come to a standstill quite some time ago.

For a long time the static nature of reliability went unquestioned, because in the knowledge and psychometric discourses in particular (see Hodges, chapter 1), reproducibility, standardized testing, and reliability measures based on internal consistency were universally accepted as sufficient assurance that assessment would be fair and trustworthy. But with the reemergence of the performance and particularly the reflection discourses in assessment—in other words, when testing became assessment again—other assessment modalities and purposes have come to the fore, and reliability in the traditional sense has lost some of its power.

In this chapter we investigate the concept of reliability (or to be more precise, the concept of universe representation) more extensively. We present some provocative new ideas, and—as we all stand on the shoulders of giants—we also revive some concepts and methods from the past that somehow seem to have dropped from sight. But first we want to consider briefly how concepts of validity have developed and discuss the relationship between validity and reliability.

Validity Theory

The most commonly used definition of validity is the extent to which a test measures what it is purported to measure. In its simplicity, this elegant definition manages to capture the complexity of assessment. It does not narrowly prescribe *what* a test should measure, it does not define validity as a dichotomy (it does not claim that a test is either valid or invalid, but always valid only up to a point), and it stresses that a test cannot be valid per se but only in relation to a specific purpose. In spite of different conceptual approaches to validity during the past century, these central tenets have stood their ground.

The original notion of validity is rooted in the idea of criterion validity; that is, does performance on a certain test predict performance on a certain criterion? This idea is intuitively appealing since many tests are used to predict future performance. In cases where (future) performance can actually be measured, criterion validity is a useful concept. We illustrate this with an example from medicine. Screening or early diagnostic tests can be useful in predicting whether someone will develop a certain disease. As the presence of many diseases can usually be determined with sufficient certainty, the predictive validity of a test is quite easy to express in terms of false-positive and false-negative test results or as predictive values.

In (medical) education, however, reliance on criterion validity is problematic, because many criteria are intangible, defying direct observation or measurement. In contrast to height, which can be observed and measured directly, intelligence, for example, can only be inferred from observed behavior or performance. Such assumed but not directly observable characteristics are called constructs. The construct validity of a test is conditional on the validity of the construct. If criterion validation were our only validation instrument, we would be forced to validate the criterion for the criterion, and so forth, leading to infinite regress.

Another intuitively appealing approach is collecting judgments as to whether a test measures the construct at hand. There are many situations in which this is defensible, especially if performance is almost identical to the characteristic to be assessed. A case in point is the ability to play a musical instrument. To assess a candidate's ability to play the flute, for example, a panel of expert judges might be asked to judge the candidate's performance of different pieces of music on different occasions. However, while judgment-based validity may be acceptable for this type of construct, its appropriateness for other human characteristics is less clear-cut, because at some stage in the validation process the observed performances will have to be translated into a construct. It is here that judges' personal beliefs and convictions come into play, self-fulfilling prophecies may cloud clear judgments, and so forth. In summary, human judgment as the sole measure of the validity of educational tests has quite serious limitations.

A crucial contribution to the development of validity theory was the paper on construct validity in which Cronbach and Meehl (1955) posited that the validation process should start from sound and defensible assumptions about the construct to be measured. Based on such assumptions it would be feasible to collect data and conduct experiments to support the validity of an assessment instrument. Let us return to the construct of "intelligence." An intelligence test cannot be validated unless we have first defined the characteristics of intelligence to be tested. These could be based on assumptions such as: intelligent people learn faster, are better able to understand abstract concepts, process information faster, have superior memory skills, and so on. Next we have to conduct different validation studies to demonstrate the validity of the intelligence test. Such studies should demonstrate, for example, that the test can differentiate between candidates, that candidates with superior memory skills also are quicker to understand abstract concepts (that is, that the different characteristics of the construct are correlated), and that there are no characteristics (age, for example) besides intelligence that offer an equally acceptable or perhaps better explanation for candidates scoring differently.

This last example also offers an excellent illustration of the notion that validation of a test must also comprise critical experiments aimed at falsifying the assumption of validity: the so-called falsification principle. Only if falsification attempts fail repeatedly will their results contribute to the validity of the test.

Since then, important work on construct validity has been done by others, such as Messick (Messick 1994). The theoretical framework of validity that is currently dominant was proposed by Kane (2006). It relies on a series of inferences linking observations of performance to a construct. A first inference is made from observation to test score, the second from test score to universe score, the third from universe score to the target domain, and the fourth from the target domain to the construct. (More inferences are thinkable depending on the circumstances, but for this chapter these four inferences suffice to explain the principle.) It is up to the researchers to provide arguments and/or to design and conduct critical studies to lend support to each of these inferences. In this way a coherent, solid bridge can be constructed connecting observations and construct.

With regard to the first inference (from observations to scores), studies could address negative marking, open-ended versus multiple-choice items, but also observer bias (see below for a medical example of validity inferences). As for the third inference, it would be appropriate to study the effects of combining results within a test (weighting), triangulation of results, and standard setting. The fourth inference could be addressed through studies of conjunctive and compensatory models, collation and judgment processes, and so forth.

An example we have used often to illustrate that in many validity situations similar inferences must be made is taking someone's blood pressure. For this, several inferences must be made as well:

- *From observation to score*: Physicians must translate what they hear through the stethoscope and see on the sphygmomanometer to a numerical value. They can make valid inferences as to the numerical value of the blood pressure only if they know which values to use, let the sphygmomanometer run down correctly, use the right cuff, etc.

- *From observed score to universe score:* But one observation is not enough; in many cases multiple ones are needed to ensure that the physician's observations are sufficiently representative of all possible observations. The Dutch guidelines, for example, state that hypertension can be diagnosed only if the blood pressure is taken twice during one consultation and this is repeated during a second consultation at least twenty-four hours later.

- *From universe score to target domain:* In order for the results of the blood pressure measurements to be used in conclusions about the cardiovascular status of the patient, heart auscultation, pulse palpation, etc., all need to be incorporated, and all results need to be triangulated.

- *From target domain to construct:* To determine the patient's health the cardiovascular status needs to be used in conjunction with other signs, symptoms, and findings; and for this, further information will be sought from other sources and needs to be triangulated to come to a comprehensive diagnosis.

Reliability is at the center of the *second* inference, hinging on the notion that a finite set of observations can support an infinite conclusion. Obviously this is not a new issue. Indeed it is a very old one in the scientific discourse. We will make a detour into the broader realm of science to refresh

our understanding of inductivism. With regard to inductivism, philosophy of science acknowledges that no matter how often an experiment is
replicated or an observation repeated, absolute certainty is unattainable, as
there is no way we can effectively exclude the possibility of a trustworthy
observation or critical experiment undermining the infinite conclusion (or
scientific law). In inductivistic science this dilemma is dealt with by formu-
lating necessary conditions—namely, that a large number of trustworthy
observations must be obtained, under a wide variety of conditions, and that
it is unacceptable for any of the observations (or statements derived from
them) to conflict with the derived law (Chalmers 1999). We also want to
call attention to one underlying assumption that is crucial but rarely made
explicit: that of natural phenomena always obeying a certain lawfulness.

Our brief excursion into inductivism may have seemed somewhat unexpected, but we only digressed to strengthen the argument we want to
make in this chapter. In a nutshell, we wish to assert that, before we can
make any claims about the credibility of inferences from observed scores
(or test results) to a universe score, it is fundamental to critically and carefully scrutinize the implicit and explicit assumptions underlying these
inferences.

By now it may have become clear that reliability and validity cannot
be regarded as two separate entities of the psychometric quality of assessment but should be seen as two concepts that are inextricably intertwined.
Reliability is not only prerequisite for validity, but—as an element of universe generalization—it is an essential step in establishing the validity of
an assessment.

Assumptions to Be Made in the Process

Using reliability as the sole underpinning of inferences from observed
scores to universe scores reflects a very narrow perspective, and the currently popular practice of using Cronbach's alpha as *the* method of choice
seems even more shortsighted. We are not alone in this opinion. Cronbach
himself in his final paper expressed regret about this development (Cronbach and Shavelson 2004). Let us briefly review some of the sacrifices we
would be forced to make in assessment if we narrowly define universe representation as reliability or reproducibility.

First, we should appreciate that any measure of internal consistency is only a proxy measure of a proxy measure for universe representation, that is, the extent to which a candidate's observed score (or the conclusions based on it) is representative of the candidate's scores on all possible items in the domain. Similarly, any real test-retest correlation is only a sample of one out of a universe of all possible real test-retest correlations. To complicate matters even further, in some situations real test-retest correlation is impossible to measure. In those cases, we have recourse to a split-half approach by randomly splitting the test into two halves, calculating the correlation between them, and correcting for test length. Clearly, the number of possible split-halves can be very high, increasing the chance of finding a correlation that is spuriously high or low. To prevent this, many different split-half correlations can be calculated—using the mean as the approximation of reliability—or the test can be split into as many parts as possible. This is the basis for internal consistency measures (such as Cronbach's alpha). Given the manner in which internal consistency is calculated, we have to conclude that its use as an indication of universe representation is conditional on the assumption of a homogeneous universe of all possible observations. That this asks for quite a leap of faith is illustrated by the following medical example. Suppose we draw blood from a patient to determine the hemoglobin level. If we homogenize the blood sample and determine the hemoglobin level of three subsamples, we would be right in expecting the same result every time. Any variance we would logically attribute to (measurement) error, because we have good reason to assume that the sample is homogeneous for hemoglobin. But if we put the blood sample in a so-called ESR column, the red cells will precipitate and be separated from the white cells (buffy coat) and the plasma. In that case we should not be surprised to find different hemoglobin levels in random subsamples. Quite the contrary in fact. If we were to find the same value for every sample, we should doubt the validity of our instrument, for we know that in our second example the "universe" from which we took the samples is not homogeneous, and it would be a grave mistake to attribute variance to measurement error.

Our reasoning so far has given us ample cause to wonder whether the automatic assumption of homogeneity might be harmful. We would argue that it often is, and we will clarify this by an example from education. An educationalist has to set the standard for an examination and decides to use an Angoff procedure. One of the eight judges on the panel consistently makes much stricter judgments than the other panel members. Worse still, she persists in her strictness after her deviant judgments have been the topic of an open and lengthy discussion between the judges. As an experienced and active teacher she is familiar with students' performance. Also, her many years of teaching experience have made her eminently knowledgeable on the subject of the examination in question. Yet her ratings are consistently and considerably higher than those of the other judges. The educationalist sees no other solution than to remove her data from the matrix (while correcting for the lower number of judges) to increase the internal consistency of the cutoff score. He logically, albeit naively, concludes that his action has increased the reliability/reproducibility of the standard-setting procedure and consequently improved the universe representation. But has it? In fact, by removing a valid element (actually 12.5%) from the sample, the educationalist is more likely to have harmed universe representation. To enhance it he would have done better to increase the number of strict judges, thereby correcting for the apparent bias toward leniency in the domain sampling (too few strict judges). We agree that this example may seem rather extreme and far-fetched. But is it really? Unfortunately, it is awfully similar to all those instances where test items are removed for no other reason than poor item statistics. And if we give it some more thought we are forced to concede that what is common practice in assessment would be rightfully called data manipulation in research. To reiterate our core argument: the assumption of homogeneity of the test universe should not be made lightly.

A second assumption about the construct to be measured is that it is stable and generic, at least for the duration of the measurement. In many traditional test situations, this is a defensible assumption. Take the example of a two-hour multiple-choice test on medical knowledge. We should expect to be accused of nit-picking if we seriously warned against the risk that the candidates' knowledge might change perceptibly during the test. However, things are different when we collect and combine the results of a series of mini clinical evaluation exercises (CEXs) collected over a three-month practice rotation. In this case the assumption of construct stability rests on less solid ground. Indeed, it would be more logical to assume that the object of measurement *does* change during the measurement period (wouldn't education be useless if we found otherwise?). Nonetheless, if we apply psychometric methods based on construct stability to longitudinal measurements, we have no other logical choice than to attribute all changes (increased competence or improved results due to learning between measurement moments) in the construct to error.

As we stated in our excursion into philosophy of science, note must be taken of the implicit but omnipresent assumption of stable lawfulness. In assessment this means that we assume that all the information about a student's test performance "adds up" to a personal characteristic that is more or less lawful. This argument may seem overly philosophical and abstract, but we will try to make it more concrete. If a medical student gives proof that he knows that oxytocin is produced by the posterior pituitary gland, there is no logical reason to infer that he also knows that surfactant is produced by type II alveolar cells. By contrast, it *would be* logical to assume that a student who clearly demonstrates that he understands the Frank-Starling mechanism—the concept that the more a heart muscle is stretched the stronger it contracts; an important underlying concept in heart failure—also understands that the heart is mainly a muscle. Both examples are concerned with the defensibility of combining test item scores. While the first example raises doubt, the second one seems more reassuring. With factual knowledge tests we are generally quite confident that it is justifiable to combine the results on different items (even across blueprint categories), but we can think of test situations where it may be less defensible. If in an objective structured clinical examination (OSCE), we combine the results on a communication station with the results on a resuscitation station, we are implicitly assuming that the OSCE is measuring some stable underlying construct. This leaves us no option but to attribute any intraindividual variance in scores to measurement error. In clinical practice, however, case-to-case variance is meaningful. It seems that in assessment we are generally acting on the overarching assumption that each test measures one stable and generic construct allowing us to combine the results of test elements that, albeit similar in format, are completely different in content (like the OSCE stations). We do so despite the abundance of evidence that correlation between test elements that are similar in content but different in format is much stronger than correlation between test elements that are different in content but similar in format (Maatsch and Huang 1986; Norman 1988; Norman et al. 1987; Norman, Swanson, and Case 1996). Translating our example to clinical practice, the OSCE example would equate to a doctor telling you that your blood glucose level is far too high and your sodium level far too low, but that you are not to worry, because on average you are in reasonably good health. In the light of the preceding argumentation, we would suggest careful (re)consideration of the frequently voiced objections to so-called core items—items in a test that are deemed so essential that any candidate answering them incorrectly should fail the whole test. The usual argument is that these items reduce reliability and should therefore not be used. But how valid is this argument considering it does not necessarily imply that core items or stations reduce universe representation?

Interestingly, there are scientific views emerging that performance evaluations should not be approached as attempts to capture a stable characteristic but as attempts to measure and predict the interaction between the candidate and the situation. In line with this approach, disciplines like situated cognition and ecological psychology do not offhandedly dismiss interaction effects as errors but value them as potentially meaningful signals.

We have now come to a third assumption, about the relationship between subjectivity and objectivity on the one hand, and reliability and unreliability on the other hand. Despite its frequent usage, the term "objectivity" should not be used lightly. Why we should be wary of casual usage of the term is explained elegantly by Alan Chalmers (1999) in his book on philosophy of science. He takes us back to the days when people were still debating whether the world was a flat object or a globe spinning in space. The killer argument would have been to jump up to demonstrate that one lands on the same spot (or that any deviations are nonsystematic). This test would lend itself to replication in many ways and many places (all around the globe). Since the result would be the same every time, it would have been the perfectly reproducible and falsifying experiment and therefore solid proof that the world is *not* a spinning globe in space. Only after the laws of inertia were discovered could it be explained why the jumping experiment was not valid. To return to assessment in education, the bottom line is that objective interpretation of test results is impossible and any test is subjective. This is certainly true for assessment of medical competence and performance: what is seen as a good doctor now was not seen as a good doctor fifty years ago, but for the present moment there is sufficient agreement about the capacities (competencies) of a good doctor. Based on this, and using human judgment and opinions, we decide what should be in the curriculum and how it should be taught. Next, we determine the content of a specific course or module and what the test should look like (these are all judgments). Finally, we set the questions and make judgments about their specific content, phrasing, and relevance. Only after completing all these—subjective—judgment processes do we capture the result in a numerical score, suddenly asserting that the test is "objective." This is hardly convincing. We want to argue here that there is no such thing as an objective test. But regardless of this, the notion that objectivity equals good universe representation and subjectivity equals poor universe representation is a harmful misrepresentation. The endeavor to "objectify" assessment into tickable items in the expectation that this will increase universe generalization has led to trivialized and mechanistic types of assessment in past decades. Fortunately, general conceptions have changed, and it is now increasingly accepted that universe generalization comes from good sampling, not from overstructuring (Van der Vleuten, Norman, and De Graaf 1991).

Approaches to Universe Generalization

In this section we want to discuss the various approaches to universe representation that we need to consider when designing and validating assessment methods or programs. We do not claim that all of this is new. Many approaches have been developed that for some reason have been forgotten or have gone out of use. We will discuss three different concepts: reproducibility, saturation, and expertise.

Reproducibility

Reproducibility is the best-known approach, and we have discussed elements of it in the previous sections. Of the various levels at which it can be determined, three are the most popular:

1. Would the student obtain the same score if s/he were to sit a parallel test?[1]

---

1. A parallel test is a hypothetical test of equal difficulty on the same topic but with other items than the original.

2. Would the rank ordering from best- to worst-performing student be the same on the parallel test?
3. Would the pass-fail decision be the same for all students on the parallel test?

In most cases these questions are addressed from a norm-oriented perspective. This means that the test is good if it is optimally able to discriminate between students, that is, to determine whether John did better than Jim. So items must not have extreme p-values and must have positive item-total or item-rest correlations (Rit or Rir, or their pendants in other psychometric theories). If a test has many zero-variance items, reliability will automatically be low (though universe representation may still be high), and if all students score all items correctly, all p-values are 1 and Rit or Rir cannot be calculated. From the perspective of a certifying body this may seem defensible, but from the viewpoint of an educational organization it is not helpful at all, because it means that if your education is perfect and all students master the relevant subject matter perfectly, there is no way you will be able to establish the quality of your tests. Apart from that, the main focus of an educational organization is not discriminating between different students but optimizing the learning effects for all students. The main question is not whether John is better than Jim, but whether today John is optimally better than he was yesterday, and the same goes for Jim (and of course whether their progress is good enough). Educational organizations therefore are best served by methods enabling them to determine the universe representation of each individual student's test score regardless of other students' scores.

It may seem strange that this issue has not been thought of before. In fact, by the mid-1960s Cronbach was already beginning to question whether classical test theory was useful for all testing situations, and authors such as Popham, Hambleton, Swaminathan, and Berk (Berk 1980; Hambleton and Novik 1973; Hambleton et al. 1978; Popham and Husek 1969; Swaminathan, Hambleton, and Algina 1974) did further work developing methods to determine reliability. These methods can be subdivided into threshold loss and squared-error loss agreement indexes. The former are based on the proportions of candidates obtaining the same mastery/non-mastery classifications on subsequent (parallel or equated) tests, while the latter are based on consistency of measurement of scores (squared deviations of individual scores from the cutting score). Both types of approaches share the disadvantage of requiring a predefined cutting score and of needing the results of a group of candidates before agreement indexes can be calculated. But they do not need firm assumptions about score distribution and they do not need candidate scores to vary per se. Theoretically, they can be applied if all candidates obtain the same results, but their values must be interpreted with caution, taking into account the cutting score, test length, and mean scores. So although these methods allow for comparison without forcing interindividual score variance, they still require scores of a group of candidates, and they are also based on the assumption that the object of measurement remains unchanged during and between test administrations.

Saturation

As we discussed above, reproducibility is based on the notion of construct stability. Whenever we seek to determine whether the results on another test are the same as the results on the current test, the underlying assumption is that what we want to measure remains stable across repeated measurements. Obviously, this is not a realistic starting point. It is logical to assume that many aspects of medical competence are not homogeneous or stable in nature, but heterogeneous and changing over time (even during the measurement). Every approach to universe generalization based on the assumption of homogeneity or stability will inevitably underestimate the universe generalization. If we go back to our earlier example of the Angoff procedure, the assumption of homogeneity would lead us to eliminate the ratings of the outlier judge. The notion of heterogeneity, on the other hand, would lead us to seek out more judges of the outlier type, adding more judges until addition no longer provides unique new information. This principle is well-known to medical practitioners; in patient care a physician will go on collecting diagnostic information until s/he is confident that any new information is unlikely to change his/her diagnostic or management decisions. This does not mean that all diagnostic information must support one single diagnosis; the principle also applies with multimorbidity (so prevalent in patient care). At the point where specifically determined new diagnostic information does not add relevant information to the complete picture of the patient, a point of saturation and—thus—universe representation has been reached.

This notion differs fundamentally from the previous one of reproducibility, in which agreement is essential (the more agreement, the better the universe representation). In the saturation approach agreement is irrelevant; what is essential is the probability of new information being relevant to the conclusion or decision. This principle is not new either. It is widely used in qualitative research. In building new theoretical models, for example, the researcher may stop collecting additional information or analyzing new transcripts when s/he has not encountered new themes or ideas for some time. There can be some debate in qualitative research as to when it is safe to say that saturation has been reached, but our main concern here is that this line of thinking creates new possibilities for assessment. An example was described by Driessen et al. (2005), who proposed a new approach to the judgment of student portfolios. Instead of forcing judges to agree by setting up a detailed scoring rubric, they designed a logistical setup with cycles of additional information gathering being repeated until no new information could be obtained. They employed all kinds of methods derived from qualitative research to guarantee universe representation while avoiding the pitfall of the trivializing checklist approach. In his overview, Berk (1980) describes several probabilistic procedures to determine the universe generalization of proportional scores on a test—in other words, whether the proportion of items answered correctly by an individual student is indicative of the proportion of correctly answered items if that student had attempted all the possible items in the domain. Such approaches are useful as they allow assessors to establish (even on the fly) whether or not saturation is reached. In 2002 (Schuwirth et al. 2002) we adopted a similar approach to evaluate the universe representation of the so-called practice performance procedures, encompassing a site visit to an individual doctor to determine his/her fitness to practice independently. This was an expensive assessment in which information from various sources (third-party interviews, lab-ordering data, chart-stimulated discussions, etc.) was collected and judged on an ordinal scale (satisfactory, doubtful, cause for concern). We used a binomial approach to determine whether it was worth the expense to continue collecting information in one domain or whether it made more sense to proceed to another source of information. The approach proved to be feasible, trustworthy, and increased the efficiency of the procedure.

These are just illustrations of what can be done and they are not intended as proof of the suitability of the method. For this, much more work needs to be done, and the illustrations and the work of Berk and his contemporaries provide a good basis for that.

Expertise

"I am an experienced assessor; I have examined students for thirty years, and one minute into an examination I know what they are worth." Any decent psychometrician or test developer will tell you that this teacher is sadly misinformed. "I am an experienced internist; I have practiced for over thirty years, and one minute after the start of a consultation I know the diagnosis." Any clinical reasoning researcher would tell you that this internist may be not so very much mistaken, because experts can make a quick diagnosis with far more accuracy than novices (Eva 2004; Regehr and Norman 1996; and see Mylopoulos, chapter 4 in this volume). Is it strange that decisions based on assessment should be so different from a diagnostic classification task? Is not the process by which examiners reach the diagnosis of "medical incompetence" largely similar to the one leading to the diagnosis of "appendicitis"? In fact, there is increasing evidence supporting the similarity of the two processes (Govaerts et al. 2007). Like diagnostic expertise, assessor expertise develops through the emergence of scripts or schemata. Expert assessors process information about the performance of a candidate at a higher interpretative level, chunking information and referring to role (what can be expected of a second-year medical student), person, and event schemata (Govaerts et al. 2011). These findings have huge implications.

A first important implication is that expert assessors should not be cast out but warmly welcomed. Human judgment should not be sacrificed on the altar of "objectivity," nor should it be "straitjacketed" into highly structured assessment formats or forms. A fortunate corollary of using expert instead of intermediate or novice assessors is the smaller sample needed to reach the same level of universe representation, simply because the "diagnosis" made by the expert is richer in information.

A second important implication is that assessor training should not be limited to a workshop on an assessment instrument. Just as we should not assume that a student knows what lab tests to order just because we have taught him how to complete a lab form, we would be very naive to assume that knowing how to complete a mini-CEX form makes a teacher an expert assessor. On-the-job training, case-exchange meetings of assessors to evaluate each other's cases and decisions, feedback, second opinions— they all belong to the training track of expert assessors. With regard to examiner training for workplace-based assessment in particular, it would be most unwise to expect a better structured test form to lead to better universe representation; there simply is no easy alternative to providing proper training for assessors. This is in accordance with the currently popular adage that the quality of structured tests (like a multiple-choice-questions paper) is built into the paper and does not depend on the expertise of the one administering the test, whereas in any observation-based assessment the paper is of minor importance but the user is essential for test quality.

Expertise development and through it better universe representation do not result from the elimination of so-called biases, but from strengthening them. In fact these biases are nothing less than strategies to reduce cognitive load (Van Merriënboer and Sweller 2005, 2010) caused by an excessive amount of information to be processed. Schemata and scripts are stereotypes as long as they are unripe, but as they mature they become increasingly powerful tools. Training should therefore be focused on furthering the development of stereotypes into mature and flexible scripts. The same applies to all kinds of other biases, such as salience effects, primacy and halo effects, fundamental attribution, and so forth. Instead of trying to reduce assessors to a "neutral window on reality," we should nurture their expertise. If training really helps enhance and enrich judgment processes, we postulate that it will improve rather than worsen universe representation, just as supporting the development of illness scripts does not lead to poorer but to better diagnoses.

Conclusion

We do not pretend to offer this chapter as a narrative review. Instead our aim has been to present ideas and opinions challenging all those involved in assessment—be it as a psychometrician, teacher, or assessment developer—to think out of the box.

In this chapter we also want to support many of the intuitive notions of experienced teachers that classical and modern test theory have been so quick to discard—notions such as core items, the relevance of situativity, the importance of student by case interaction, and the role of assessor expertise—mainly because we think that the dominance of psychometric theories in guiding our thinking about quality of assessment and its resulting decisions has been far too one-sided.

Our purpose in writing this chapter was therefore to help readers see more clearly that there are many ways of approaching the argument around the generalization of a limited set of observations in assessment to a universe of all possible observations and that we have at our disposal a plethora of methods, concepts, and instruments. Whether all of these will prove useful is debatable. But a one-size-fits-all-practice approach to universe generalization (even at the conceptual level) is no longer tenable—of that we are quite certain.

Blinded by "Insight"

Self-Assessment and Its Role in Performance Improvement

Kevin W. Eva, Glenn Regehr, and Larry D. Gruppen

> Beware the Jabberwock, my son!
> The jaws that bite, the claws that catch!
> Beware the Jubjub bird, and shun
> The frumious Bandersnatch!
>
> Lewis Carroll, *Through the Looking Glass*

In Carroll's *Through the Looking Glass* Alice discovers a poem, "Jabberwocky," that can be read only when held up to a mirror. So too have many others suggested that we as individuals can read ourselves only through deliberate acts of reflection. Among professionals ranging from athletic coaches to business leaders, there is a general belief that the path to better performance is through "looking in the mirror" to openly and honestly identify one's weaknesses and take steps to improve them. As a result, many models of professional self-regulation worldwide and many health professional training curricula have incorporated some form of planned self-assessment activity into their practices (Sargeant et al. 2010). In fact, the health professions may provide the most extreme example, as their current models of maintenance of competence and self-regulation are formalizations, in large part, of the instruction "Physician, know thyself." Generally, the practitioner is expected to reflect on his or her performance (preferably by incorporating indicative evidence) and to determine an appropriate course of action to ensure self-directed learning and maintenance of competence (Handfield-Jones et al. 2002). This expectation has prompted an industry of research into self-assessment and related constructs that has yielded both data and a reaction reminiscent of Alice's after she has read the poem. "'It seems very pretty,' she said when she had finished it, 'but it's rather hard to understand!' (You see she didn't like to confess, even to herself, that she couldn't make it out at all.) 'Somehow it seems to fill my head with ideas—only I don't exactly know what they are!'"

Debate regarding the extent to which self-assessment can or should play a central role in the regulatory efforts and competency frameworks of the health professions has amplified in recent years (Eva and Regehr 2005). Most of it has centered around whether individuals are inherently incapable of judging the strength of their abilities or whether such judgments tend to correlate poorly with externally derived measures because individuals need to learn how to be reflective, how to incorporate external feedback into their self-perceptions, and what the community's standards are with respect to performance expectations. Debate at this level implies that the fundamental challenge in the notion of self-regulation resides in the ability of individuals to perceive performance deficiencies accurately. Unquestionably we each have more information available to us with which to judge our own abilities than do any external observers. It is this very wealth of information, however, that may prevent us from generating accurate impressions of our own abilities. Our research and that of others raises questions about the adequacy of self-assessment, reasons why inadequate self-assessment may actually be adaptive, and the many ways in which we can fool ourselves into believing that we have privileged insight into our own capacities. This research raises fundamental concerns about the way in which the health professions typically conceive of self-assessment and the purposes for which it can be applied in a productive manner. Further, it is becoming increasingly clear that even if individuals were readily able to identify strengths and weaknesses in their performance, there are other issues that must be considered to determine the extent to which individuals can be expected to use perceived deficits to guide performance improvements (Regehr and Eva 2006; Regehr and Mylopoulos 2008).

In this chapter we examine the foundations of many modern theories of self-improvement, lay and otherwise, raising fundamental concerns about how health professions typically conceive of and apply self-assessment. We conclude the chapter with a description of how models of professional self-regulation can be effectively modified given the evidence base that has accumulated to date.

Laying the Groundwork

> If you wanna make the world a better place,
> take a look at yourself and then make a change.
>
> Michael Jackson, "Man in the Mirror"

Judgments of personal competence underlie everything we do, and the notion that we can improve ourselves (and the world) by more carefully considering the "person in the mirror" is prevalent. We make judgments about our competence whenever we decide that we are able to navigate the streets in a strange city rather than rely on the support of professional taxi drivers, whenever we apply for a promotion to a job that we consider ourselves capable of doing, or whenever we initiate a treatment regimen for patients we consider ourselves knowledgeable or skilled enough to help. Through these examples it can be seen that the stakes of inaccurate self-assessment vary and that the decision not to act when one has the capacity can be as costly as the decision to act when one should not. Within the health professions it has largely become universal that the onus of responsibility for the maintenance of competence is placed on the individual practitioner. In scanning the revalidation and recertification policies of eighteen countries, Peck et al. (2000, 435), concluded that "approaches differ widely around the world, but most rely on professional self-regulation." As such, it is imperative that we understand the limits of the various activities related to maintenance of competence and professional development, including our ability to self-assess.

It would seem self-evident that each of us, as individuals, has greater opportunity to generate insights into the strengths and limits of our own performance and ability than does anyone else. There must be tremendous insight to be gained from total knowledge of one's past experiences (as opposed to the samples available to external observers), awareness of the motivations leading us to act in certain ways, and the inner thoughts that others have access to only to the extent that we choose to (or can) share them. This notion is so self-evident and the intuition so powerful that we readily and commonly attribute flaws in others to lack of self-awareness; we easily discount information received from other sources as being noncredible (e.g., resulting from inadequate observation, personality conflicts, or invalid testing protocols); and we routinely present improved self-reflection as a mechanism to guide performance improvements. Any one of these interpretations will be correct in some circumstances, but the important issue is the proportion of times in which they are correct. As we have written before, accurately knowing that one could never play professional football is not an argument for accurate self-assessment because one needs also to consider how frequently we are inaccurate in "knowing" we are able to (or could not) perform certain tasks well (Eva and Regehr 2008).

Before getting into these issues in greater detail, however, it is crucially important to clearly and explicitly define the terms we will use to consider the issues we hope to address because we are convinced that the implicit nature of these definitions in many conversations has yielded considerable confusion and conflict. We make no claim that these are the only ways in which the following terms could be used, but they are definitions that have helped us conceptualize critical distinctions between aspects of cognition and models of self-regulation that are often confounded in the health professions education literature. Furthermore, we think it critical that the community come to some form of agreed-on taxonomy to lessen the communication difficulties, misunderstandings, and derivation of inappropriate implications that can arise from loose use of language.

Consistent with our earlier work, we will define *self-assessment* as a personal, unguided reflection on performance for the purposes of generating an individually derived summary judgment of one's own level of knowledge, skill, and understanding in a particular area (Eva and Regehr 2008). There are several aspects of this definition that we consider important to highlight. First, in this definition we have framed self-assessment as a process, not as the outcome of that process. We think this distinction is important because the failure to make this distinction has been one of the major sources of confusion in the community's discussions. Several authors have suggested, for example, that manipulations that bring self-assessment scores in line with objectively derived scores are an indicator that they have "improved self-assessment." Yet this interpretation is problematic. Since most people tend to overassess their performance, improving actual performance tends to bring actual scores more in line with self-assessment scores (Kruger and Dunning 1999, study 4). However, this incidental alignment of self-assessed and actual scores does not imply an improvement in the process of self-assessment any more than moving a target to where someone is throwing a ball implies that we are improving their aim. Thus, we feel it important to distinguish *self-assessment* the verb from *self-assessment* the noun. Unfortunately, we have as yet found no sensible set of labels that readily enables this distinction; so we will simply highlight the issue here and, throughout this chapter, try to be explicit about whether we are describing the process of self-assessment or the outcome of that process.

Second, self-assessment as we have defined it is distinct from issues of *self-concept* (Cervone 2000) in that self-assessment involves an element of context-specific appraisal rather than simply indicating how one self-identifies. Relative to self-concept, self-assessment, in the way we define it, is more immediate and transient rather than a longer-term stable construction of our self-worth. As a result, the construct of self-assessment better aligns with *self-efficacy,* the domain-specific belief in one's capabilities to perform in a certain manner (Cervone 2000). In the social psychology literature, self-efficacy is spoken of as a determinant of performance in addition to being a judgment of one's ability (i.e., positive self-efficacy can yield better performance relative to negative self-efficacy; see Dweck 1999). Outside of that literature, however, self-assessment is more generally spoken of simply in terms of reflecting one's capability and, as a result, while we think the bidirectional aspect of self-appraisal and performance is important, we will treat the terms *self-assessment* and *self-efficacy* separately.

Third, the "individually derived" portion of our definition of self-assessment stands in stark contrast to the definitions offered by Boud (1999) and by Epstein, Siegel, and Silberman (2008), who argued that self-assessment should be conceived of as self-appraisal derived from the interaction between internally derived perceptions and externally generated data regarding the strength of one's performance or abilities. We do not deny that such interactions are important and, indeed, we presume that self-assessments are always informed to some extent by one's experienced successes and failures. However, we have included the concept "individually derived" in our definition for two reasons. First, much of the research addressing self-assessment has implicitly used this concept in the operational definition. That is, most studies attempt to measure self-assessment ability by having participants engage in some performance, assessing that performance, asking participants to make their own summary assessment of the performance, then comparing the externally derived assessments to the individually derived assessments. We believe that the ubiquity of this "guess your grade" model of self-assessment research (and its implied assumptions about the process) both reflects and reinforces an implicit model of the self-assessment process that leans heavily on a belief that people can determine for themselves their level of performance and ability. Second, we believe that important cognitive processing takes place at the intersection between one's self-perceptions and the interpretation of external data (as will be discussed below). This processing is heavily determined by factors beyond the data on which the self-assessment process is purportedly based. Thus, we will use the term *informed self-assessment* (Sargeant et al. 2010) to refer to Boud's and Epstein, Siegel, and Silberman's versions of self-assessment as a deliberately interactive process of incorporating data available from the environment into one's self-assessment. In this way, informed self-assessment is related to *self-directed assessment seeking* (Eva and Regehr 2008), the pedagogical activity of intentionally looking outward for formative and summative assessments of one's current levels of performance.

Finally, we note that the definition of self-assessment as resulting in a "summary judgment" of one's ability in a particular area invokes a crucial distinction between broader judgments of how well one performs in an area generally and how one determines, *in the moment,* whether or not one is performing in a way that is yielding the outcomes one desires (what we have referred to in previous work as *self-monitoring;* Eva and Regehr 2007, 2011). That is, as a broad judgment, self-assessment might be used as a mechanism through which to self-limit one's decisions about general domains of practice (e.g., "I no longer accept referrals for those types of cases"). As a much more narrow level of judgment, self-monitoring can be used, in the moment, to determine whether one needs help with a particular task (e.g., "I should consult my colleague about the implications of that test result"). In this way self-assessment and self-monitoring align well with the reflective discourse identified by Hodges in chapter 1 and Schön's (1983) notions of reflection-on-practice and reflection-in-practice, respectively. We have opted not to adopt these terms because *reflection* is a broader notion in that it has also been used (in much of the expertise literature, for example) to describe the act of investing mental energy into understanding "why" the world works in the way it does rather than simply as a mechanism through which to judge personal competence (Mann, Gordon, and MacLeod 2009).

Direct Tests of Self-Assessment

> You're on your own. And you know what you know.
> And YOU are the guy who will decide where to go.
>
> DR. SEUSS, *Oh, the Places You'll Go!*

In 1962 the American Medical Association and Association of American Medical Colleges issued a joint report that declared, "Self-appraisal is a test which each of us has applied to himself for so long that we hardly consider the matter" (Gordon 1991, 762). Since then hundreds of studies have been conducted to "consider the matter," and their results have generally led to the conclusion that, perhaps for the only time, Dr. Seuss was wrong: people do not seem to "know what they know." In one of the first reviews on the topic within the health professions, Gordon (ibid.) summarized the literature up to 1990: "The validity of self-assessed performance was found to be low to moderate and did not improve with time in conventional health professions training programs. Self-assessed performance seemed closely related to generalized self-attributions and was minimally influenced by external feedback in the form of test scores, grades, or faculty assessments." This damning conclusion did not curb the optimism Gordon expressed regarding the potential to create effective interventions to overcome this problem (1992), but despite two decades of additional research, the conclusions of many others are consistently bleak.

Because the literature has been reviewed many times (see Davis et al. 2006, for an example focused on self-assessment among practicing physicians), we will not provide a comprehensive review here. That said, the pattern of findings can be summarized fairly concisely: an investigator team reports a poor correlation between self-assessment and external performance data; subsequent investigators identify methodological weaknesses and run a new study prior to reporting the same poor correlations;

repeat. To be clear, this representation of the literature is not a criticism of others as we each spent considerable time and effort on this treadmill (Eva et al. 2004; Ward, Gruppen, and Regehr 2001). The phenomenon of a poor correlation between self-rated performance and other forms of assessment is as robust as the intuition that we are able to self-assess, and therefore as a community we seem to have concluded that the data must be wrong. Yet inaccurate self-assessment has been shown across many domains, both within and outside the health professions (Dunning, Heath, and Suls 2004). There is variability in the strength of the correlations observed (Ward, Gruppen, and Regehr 2001), but no more than one would expect of any normal distribution. There is some indication that correlations can be improved with intensive feedback (yielding Gordon's optimism), but these generally appear more indicative of individuals being able to learn about weaknesses in a particular performance rather than improved capacity for accurate self-assessment (Eva 2001). More fundamentally, it is fair to question whether such correlational studies adequately represent the construct of self-assessment as opposed to a capacity to "guess your grade" (Colliver, Verhulst, and Barrows 2005). In fact, it is studies that deviate from this norm that have perhaps been most informative in yielding understanding of the difficulties inherent in judging oneself.

In a landmark study that won an Ig Nobel Prize in 2000 for "research that first makes people laugh and then makes people think," Kruger and Dunning (1999) demonstrated that those who are unskilled in a particular task (e.g., grammar and composition) have what amounts to a perceptual blindness to the aspects of the task that define skilled performance. Participants of all skill levels generally rated themselves as above average, thereby reproducing the common phenomenon that we tend to believe we perform better than most in socially desirable domains (commonly referred to as the Lake Wobegon effect), underestimate how long it will take us to complete tasks, and are overconfident in our judgments and predictions (Dunning, Heath, and Suls 2004). When participants were offered feedback via exposure to the test responses of a handful of their colleagues, those who performed particularly well on the grammar test (and tended to somewhat underestimate their ability) were able to recognize the divergence between their perceptions and reality as evidenced by their raising the ratings they gave their performance.

More important, however, is that those who performed particularly poorly (and tended to considerably overestimate their ability) were unable to take advantage of this additional information and did not alter their self-ratings. In other words, even though their colleagues demonstrated better grammar, poor performers did not recognize this fact. A later study presented in the same article demonstrated that intervening to improve performance (i.e., giving participants the skill) did improve the alignment between self-assessment and actual performance because the latter rose to meet the former. The main findings from this work have been replicated in a clinical setting focused on communication skills performance during an objective structured clinical examination (OSCE) (Hodges, Regehr, and Martin 2001).

Contrary to much of the rhetoric within the health professions, these findings suggest that the path to improved performance is directed training and feedback, not better self-assessment. Further, they also force us to recognize that alignment between self-ratings and actual performance does not necessarily derive from capacity to self-assess. Finally, the results remind us of the ever-present phenomenon of context specificity in that the extent to which one can self-assess well appears to be strongly context bound (Eva 2003; Fitzgerald, White, and Gruppen 2003). We assess ourselves accurately in domains in which we have skill/knowledge, but not in domains in which we do not. Unfortunately (or perhaps fortunately, for reasons that will be presented later), the implication is that we have no way of knowing for ourselves when we are in one state or the other.

Enough evidence has accumulated in both laboratory settings and the real world that is supportive of the argument that one cannot rely exclusively on self-perceptions of performance or ability that we will not belabor that point any further (Dunning, Heath, and Suls 2004). Instead, we turn our attention here to research aimed at fleshing out what to do with this information. Before doing so, however, it is worth explicitly noting that we have deliberately selected the pronouns "we" and "us" throughout this chapter when discussing difficulties with self-assessment. Because we are fans of irony, one of our favorite results from this entire domain of study is that people tend to believe they are less prone to bias in their self-assessment than they believe their peers to be (Friedrich 1996; Pronin, Lin, and Ross 2002). Poor self-assessment is not just a medical student problem, it is not just a health professional problem, and it is certainly not just someone else's problem; it impacts all of us in every aspect of our daily activities. As a result, determining what to do about the findings that have accumulated to date in this domain is not straightforward. The very difficulties inherent in internalizing the counterintuitive position that our self-assessments are flawed can cause us to be blinded by the insights they provide, thereby making it difficult to fully use the external information made available to us.

The Psychological Mechanisms Influencing Self-Assessment and Our Belief in It

> It would seem to me
> I remember every single...thing I know.
>
> THE TRAGICALLY HIP, "At the Hundredth Meridian"

We believe the reason so much time and energy has been devoted to grappling with issues of self-assessment and the role it should play in professional self-regulation is that it is so highly counterintuitive that one would struggle to self-assess accurately and so seemingly easy to attribute difficulties with others to their lack of this capacity. As a species, we may not readily *admit* our flaws to others, but surely we are *aware* of them at some fundamental level. And if we are not, does that not shake the very core of who we are as humans? Thoughts resonate in our heads, we can logically reason our way from one state to another, and we can plan and defend our actions. How could we be unaware of the limits of our ability when we are so seemingly capable of sophisticated introspection? Well, what if that belief in our ability to self-assess (and, more generally, to introspect—see Bargh and Chartrand 1999) was just a by-product (i.e., an epiphenomenon) of the way we've been wired to think about the world? We do not wish to become overly philosophical in raising these questions, but they speak to the very root of what the field is trying to accomplish whenever suggestions are made that improving self-assessment is a means toward the ends of better lifelong learning, maintenance of competence, and patient safety.

Close your eyes for a moment and think about yourself driving. If you are like most people, you have just thought of a reasonably relaxed experience with few of the details that determine the success of one's driving in the real world. Was the weather bad? Were there distractions present at the side of the road? Was there something playing on the radio that may have drawn your attention from your mirrors? We could go on, but the general point is that when asked to think of ourselves performing a task, we tend to think of the gist rather than the details even though it is the detail that will determine our success (Vallone et al. 1990). Furthermore, the easier it is to think of a scenario, the more likely we are to perceive that scenario as representing a probable state of affairs (Tversky and Kahneman 1973). Even the worst drivers more often than not get from point A to point B without disastrous consequences. Every time they do it makes it more likely that they will both infer from their driving record and the overall sense of safety derived from their reconstructed memories of driving that they are capable drivers and have difficulty understanding how anyone else, without this accumulation of evidence, could rightly pass negative judgment on their skill level. In other words, the "insight" derived from these past experiences simultaneously blinds us to our ability level and our capacity to judge our ability level. A trial judge may gain great confidence, over her years on the bench, in her ability to recognize liars because of the many times she has had to make these distinctions, but given that few who stand trial ever admit that they really were lying, on what basis is she deciding that her earlier judgments were accurate? Consistent with this idea, in a series of focus groups, we have heard health professionals talk about how their amount of experience determines their feelings of confidence with little to no mention of the quality of those experiences (Eva et al. 2011). A large variety of studies from the medical education and the social psychology literatures have suggested that others are better able to predict any number of things about us than we are able to predict about ourselves, including the likelihood of passing examinations (Risucci, Tortolani, and Ward 1989) and the length of our romantic relationships (MacDonald and Ross 1999), further suggesting that the extra information we have available to us about ourselves creates an illusion that we have privileged access to knowledge of our ability level.

But why would such errors in judgment be maintained? As a general rule people do not like to make mistakes or to be ignorant, and they tend to want to take action to overcome such states. Indeed, this tendency to want to "fix the problem" has led many to propose the need to create curricula and teaching strategies aimed at improving the accuracy of self-assessment. We consider this response misguided. Gilbert and Wilson (2000) coined the term "psychological immune system" as a way of describing the many cognitive mechanisms that protect us from threatening information. As with our biological immune system, the idea is that, within limits, we are better off maintaining an optimistic outlook on our ability and a "rose colored" self-concept. This is well documented in the psychology and psychiatry literature, where it is an accepted finding that depressed people appear to have a more realistic perception of their importance, reputation, locus of control, and abilities than those who are not depressed (Alloy and Abramson 1979), a phenomenon well enough established to have acquired the label "depressive realism" (Dobson and Franche 1989). As a result, we have built-in mechanisms to counteract external hazards that make us vulnerable (see Nussbaum and Dweck 2008). When we encounter information that contradicts our positive preconceptions about ourselves we have a tendency to automatically and unconsciously discount that information by blaming our car accident, for instance, on the rain, discounting the health risks inherent in our behaviors as being overblown by bad science, or blaming our poor performance on a headache or distractions created by our personal circumstances (Eva et al. 2011; Gilovich 1991; Tavris and Aronson 2007). Again, these interpretations will sometimes be accurate, but they become problematic when they are overly reflexive—though, ironically, such reflexivity may be a good thing.

This tendency may be fortunate because the self-efficacy literature leads to the conclusion that self-assessments are not simply reflections of performance. Instead, they should be thought of as fundamental determinants of performance as there is an important reciprocity between self-efficacy and success. Such beliefs are based on a variety of experimental studies that have demonstrated that randomly lowering self-efficacy can result in performance deficits relative to participants who have their self-efficacy raised by praise (Cervone 2000). Importantly, however, the type of praise matters. For example, Carol Dweck's (1999) work has illustrated that praising students for their effort yields greater long-term gain than praising students for their intelligence; those praised for their intelligence will more readily give up on a difficult task than the former group because they infer that they have reached the limit of their ability rather than perceiving a need to try harder. Implicit understandings of the value of positive self-efficacy are present throughout the professional identity literature in which individuals speak of the importance of feeling autonomous and confident in their own abilities. Many theorists argue that taking on the identity of the profession is as fundamental an aspect of competence as are the knowledge and skills associated with the profession (Lave and Wenger 1991; Mann 2011; Monrouxe 2010). Similarly, we have recently noted in focus groups conducted with health professional trainees and practitioners that participants feel a sometimes paralyzing tension between knowing they need feedback to improve and fearing information that disconfirms their practice (Mann et al. 2011).

In summary, the empirical findings surrounding self-assessment and the context-/content-specific nature of its accuracy suggest that we cannot create good self-assessors. Further, the data shedding light on the psychological mechanisms for poor self-assessment and the derived theoretical perspectives that highlight the value of confidence suggest that we should not even try. This perspective is fundamentally at odds with the prevalent notion that we need to improve self-assessment in order to enable learners and practitioners to improve performance. Rather, we would argue that we can have the greatest impact on self-assessment by ignoring it and focusing instead on ways in which we can enable individuals to develop the habits of seeking trustworthy feedback, acting on it without allowing it to become a personal threat, and enabling others to share such feedback in a way that facilitates its use.

Challenges Inherent in Trying to Inform One's Self-Assessment

> It is impossible for anyone to begin to learn that which he
> thinks he already knows.
>
> EPICTETUS, *Discourses*

The argument that improved self-assessment does not offer a mechanism through which one can appropriately limit one's practice or guide performance improvements is not an argument against the use of self-assessment. On the contrary, we think the latter argument to be a waste of breath, as the speed and automaticity of the self-assessment process is as natural and difficult to overcome as breathing itself (and, indeed, what else would we use in its stead?). In fact we have found that, on balance, individuals' self-appraisals have a greater impact on their generation of learning goals than does the external feedback they receive (Eva et al. 2010). During an OSCE established for the dual purposes of assessing student performance and offering an educational opportunity by enabling students to be observed and receive direct and immediate feedback on their clinical performance, the investigators asked students to evaluate the quality of the feedback they received and to appraise their own skill. After the OSCE, participants were asked to generate a list of learning goals and learning activities they identified as important for their continuing professional development that resulted from their experience in particular OSCE stations. The self-appraisals, quality of feedback ratings, and observer assessments (among other variables) were then submitted to a regression analysis to determine which factors, personal or external, most influenced students' generation of learning goals. The informed self-assessments that were generated by the students themselves were far and away the strongest determinant of learning goal generation, with the opinions of the raters regarding the strength of the students' performance having little effect. These findings reinforce the notion that external feedback is never delivered in a vacuum and that, as such, it is crucial to understand the context of what the learner believes about his/her own performance if one hopes to motivate the learner to receive and use any feedback provided.

As a result, the challenge of enabling performance improvements becomes even more daunting in that calls to establish mechanisms for delivering data to the individual, while valuable, often fail to recognize the difficulty inherent in overriding the strongly formed opinions we all hold about our strengths and weaknesses. The medical education world and knowledge translation industry have expended considerable energy and resources to develop audit and feedback strategies that examine physician practice patterns and provide feedback reports that indicate how one's practice aligns absolutely with formal professional guidelines or relative to a distribution of one's colleagues (Foy et al. 2005). The results of such efforts have been highly variable, in part because they generally treat the delivery of feedback as a dispassionate exercise in which the recipient is a disinterested observer whose only emotional investment is a desire to get better. We do not doubt for a second that every health professional (save, perhaps, a few notable exceptions) has a genuine desire to perform well, but we do think it important to recognize that being told one can improve inevitably carries the implication (if not more) that one has been performing at a suboptimal level. Is it any wonder then that people are more likely to believe data that suggest they are performing well relative to data that suggest they are not?

Sargeant et al. (2003), in a study of the uptake of feedback provided in the context of a physician-oriented multisource feedback exercise, found that participants' agreement with the scores assigned to them by their colleagues were positively correlated with the mean of those scores. That is, the higher we are rated, the more readily we believe the rating. Boehler et al. (2006), in a randomized controlled trial comparing different forms of feedback, illustrated that students gave higher teacher ratings when they received complimentary feedback, relative to when the feedback was constructively critical, despite finding greater performance gains in the latter group. When faced with the cognitive dissonance induced by the competing ideas that one is performing well and that one needs to improve, something has to give. It is much easier, given the psychological immune system, to poke holes in the external data provided (my tutor doesn't like me; my practice is different; that was just a fluke) than it is to decide that one's self-perceptions are flawed. Again, this argument is not put forward to say that such reasoning is always wrong, but is meant simply to draw attention to the notion that the more incongruent external data are with one's perceptions of reality, the more likely one is to simply ignore or actively discount the data.

Sometimes the tensions created by the cognitive dissonance inherent in the act of informing self-assessment are explicit and easily recognizable. For example, Kennedy et al. (2009) report that individuals feel tension between the desire to learn and concern about looking incompetent, thereby making people reluctant to seek feedback. Mann et al. (2011), in a study of physicians, medical students, and midwifery students, report similar findings and note further that individuals often struggle between wanting to deliver genuine and beneficial feedback while being hesitant to do so out of fear of damaging relationships. We suspect awareness of the emotionally evocative nature of feedback drives this tension. At other times, however, the tensions are felt and resolved much less consciously, further reinforcing the difficulty we have with knowing when we are right in discounting external information and when we are wrong to do so.

The social cognition literature presents the notion of "cold cognition," the limitations of memory and attention that can lead us to reinterpret data for the sake of reconciling it with our established view of the world even in the absence of the shock or grief that may arise when negative data that conflict with our worldview are presented (Eva et al. 2011). As examples, gamblers are known to interpret their losses as "near wins" (Gilovich 1991), and family physicians have been seen to attribute poor performance to extenuating circumstances like headaches while readily attributing good performances to their own ability (Eva et al. 2011). The universality of these sorts of discounting mechanisms and the resilience of our impressions indicate that we cannot simply tell people to be more open to external information or to collect data that will inform their self-assessments any more than we can successfully tell people to not be biased in their decision making. As regulatory authorities exist that are responsible for ensuring professional accountability, they can certainly mandate that people participate in some sort of reflective activity and members of the profession will go through the motions (Hays and Gay 2011). However, if we are to hope that the provision of data will influence performance, thereby fulfilling the formative purpose that self-assessment advocates suggest is paramount, then we need to determine how to create authentic activities that will inform individuals about how to improve without expecting to do so through an improved capacity to self-assess.

Where Do We Go from Here?

> Now, in order to answer the question, "Where do we go from here?" which is our theme, we must first honestly recognize where we are now.
> MARTIN LUTHER KING, "Where Do We Go from Here?"

It is not lost on us that to this point in the text we have likely raised problems more than we have provided solutions. This approach was felt necessary, however, because there are no simple solutions; because many of the solutions that can be proposed fall prey to the same cognitive constraints as the intuition that we can self-assess; and, as Dr. King said, because it is important to understand where we are now if we are to determine where we go from here. Given the theme of the discussion so far, it is presumably clear that we do not think we can "honestly recognize where we are now" when left to our own devices, but we have attempted to present samples of data from a variety of literatures to make three fundamental arguments:

1. The accuracy of self-assessment as an introspective process is too context dependent to be a trustworthy guide to performance improvement.

2. The inability to accurately self-assess our own weaknesses is adaptive in that the resulting optimism promotes tenacity and pushes personal and professional performance beyond the point that may be reasonable based on one's actual competence.

3. The same cognitive processes that impede the accuracy of self-assessment (and create a belief in our capacity to self-assess) prevent us from simply adopting external data when it conflicts with our self-assessment. This dynamic thereby limits the likely impact of simply informing self-assessment through the presentation of external data.

These three arguments lead us to the position that although we cannot trust self-assessment, we should encourage it as a way for peers and educators to discern how to deliver feedback in a manner that will allow receptivity and performance change. While that is not a guaranteed solution, we are led toward the view that feedback must be delivered from a position of understanding the recipients' perspective to avoid it being so incongruent that it falls on deaf ears. It must also be delivered from a position of understanding that feedback inherently creates a threat to the individual. For these reasons, we argue below that the best we can do as educators and regulatory authorities is to create opportunities for individuals to discover ways in which their performance can be improved rather than divining strategies to directly alter self-assessment as a mechanism for performance improvement. In this final section we will elaborate on these points by constructing our best guess at how models of professional self-regulation and performance improvement can be effectively modified given the evidence base that has accumulated to date. This section, however, is necessarily more speculative than those that preceded it and, as a result, should be read more as a series of ideas and research findings we think to be important for moving us forward, rather than as a fully refined model.

While the notions of informed self-assessment and the need to separate self-assessment and performance improvement lead us to the literature on feedback interventions, that literature has been developing for over a century (Brand and Stratton 1905), making it impossible for us to provide a comprehensive review within the confines of this chapter. Fortunately, good reviews exist (Archer 2010; Hattie and Timperley 2007; Kluger and DeNisi 1996; Kluger and van Dijk 2010; Shute 2008) that have highlighted intriguing findings to help further our discussion of the integration of individuals' self-assessment and external feedback. In a comprehensive meta-analysis, Kluger and DeNisi found that, contrary to the accepted wisdom that feedback is a good thing, the more threatening feedback is to the recipient's self-concept, the more likely it is to have a negative impact on performance.

These findings are consistent with Dweck's (1999) data in that being able to attribute failure to insufficient effort would seem less of an affront to one's self-concept than being faced with the prospect that failure indicates the limits of one's intellectual capacity. Furthermore, the findings suggest a mechanism through which one can understand the relative impact of qualitative versus quantitative feedback provision that was illustrated by Butler (1987). In a randomized controlled trial, Butler presented feedback to individuals in one of three forms: quantitative (i.e., marks), qualitative (i.e., comments), or both together. Not surprisingly, given the literature illustrating the inadequacy of self-assessment, constructive criticism offered in the form of qualitative commentary yielded greater learning gains than did numerical feedback; if one cannot self-assess then one cannot determine how to do better based on a number alone. More interesting, however, was that participants given both quantitative and qualitative feedback subsequently improved only at the rate of those given quantitative feedback in isolation. While these findings have yet to be replicated in the health professions, they (along with other empirical results) led Kluger and DeNisi to conclude that feedback that draws attention to cues about where one stands in relation to others, thus threatening the self, is more likely to be detrimental than feedback that does not. That said, our personal experience suggests that students desire knowledge of their grade. How this tension can be resolved is yet to be determined.

One excellent example of how data might be used to enhance performance while effectively circumventing summative self-evaluations has been offered by Galbraith, Hawkins, and Holmboe (2008) in their description of the potential use of electronic patient records (EPRs) to improve practice. As they describe, if EPRs were structured as a relational database, it would be possible for a practitioner to, for example, identify all diabetic patients in her practice who are not well controlled (e.g., all patients with HbA1c levels of greater that 6.5%). The physician might then use this knowledge to make a concerted effort to target these patients and get their diabetes under control. If the physician were not sure how to accomplish this, she might seek specific information, making effective use of the self-monitoring process of "knowing when to look it up" (Eva and

Regehr 2007) to accomplish this specific task. By engaging in this process, the physician will have improved her practice and learned about diabetes management in the process, without ever having had to engage in the summative self-assessment process of deciding she was below average (or below standard) in her ability to manage diabetes. Similarly, informative but relatively nonthreatening data can be derived from peer consultation: Mann et al. (2011) report that physicians involved in peer-oriented professional development groups value the opportunity to learn from the experiences presented in conversation between others without having to directly reconcile the belief that they are practicing well (or the desire to present an impression of practicing well) with information that indicates a gap in one's practice habits.

As a complicating factor, however, Kluger and van Dijk (2010) have demonstrated, using Higgins's self-regulation theory (1997), that negative feedback (e.g., failing to perform a task) is generally more efficacious than positive feedback when one is engaged in activity that requires avoiding a negative outcome (prevention), whereas the reverse is true when one is engaged with an activity that requires achieving a positive outcome (promotion). For example, they argue that a surgeon performing a routine procedure will be in prevention focus (i.e., with no real challenge given the surgeon's skill level, the task is largely one of avoiding mistakes). Success in this orientation is a low arousal condition resulting in little learning or alteration of behavior, whereas failure leads to stress, high arousal, and a greater influence of the (negative) feedback received. In contrast, the surgeon who is trying to perform a very novel and complicated procedure with little chance of success will be rewarded and influenced by feedback much more when a positive outcome occurs than she will be from the frustration that will arise from failing at a task that was not necessarily expected to be successful. In fact, these patterns are epitomized in several aphorisms from the clinical world such as "Big cases, big complications," which imply that there are times when negative outcomes are not surprising and therefore do not constitute a meaningful source of feedback. Of particular interest for our current purposes, Kluger and van Dijk note that an individual's orientation in complicated domains like the health professions is anything but static. Across tasks, over the course of time (and, we would add, even within a particular surgery), one's orientation may sway from performance oriented to prevention oriented and back again.

As such, one cannot assume that any particular feedback delivery strategy will universally improve performance, an argument that is reinforced both by the influence of contextual factors seen in formal feedback intervention studies (Shute 2008) and by recent arguments put forward against algorithmic (and, as a result, often inauthentic) strategies for feedback delivery (Voyer and Pratt 2011).

Consistent with this notion that feedback must be tailored to the specifics of the situation (and, more generally, that context impacts on learning, as outlined by Mylopoulos in chapter 4), a review of the literature on the effectiveness of students' evaluations of teachers led Marsh and Roche (1997) to conclude that augmenting feedback with consultation (i.e., having someone help the recipient work through the feedback received) is one of the most influential variables with respect to inducing behavior change. These findings could indicate an important distinction between "data" as information we are left to our own devices to interpret and "feedback" as meaning that is co-constructed through social interaction. If we believe Kruger and Dunning's (1999) argument that being unskilled and unaware go hand in hand, then it follows that counsel from a peer or supervisor may be necessary to help one understand (let alone determine how to use) external data when they are available. Such a counselor can help us place data in context (as guidance on how to improve performance rather than as a statement about our worth as individual practitioners), can minimize the risk of reflexively rejecting data that do not fit our preconceptions by offering alternative interpretations, and can provide a sense of accountability that will make it more difficult to simply ignore pieces of data that might fit uncomfortably within our current worldview.

It is important to note, however, that the credibility of the person giving feedback and the relationship between the person giving feedback and the recipient are likely to be important components of the process. When we interviewed individuals who were selected based on their engagement with formal informed self-assessment activities, we repeatedly heard statements suggesting that perceptions of beneficence and nonmaleficence (i.e., having good intentions towards the recipient) are important determinants of individuals' receptivity to the feedback provided by others (Eva et al. 2011). That said, the strength of one's relationship can be a double-edged sword, creating a greater opportunity for the feedback that is delivered to be seen as credible (and delivered in the recipients' best interest) while also creating a tension in that a preexisting relationship can make it less likely that feedback will be delivered for fear of damaging the relationship itself (Mann et al. 2011).

Fortunately, guidance exists regarding ways in which situations might be constructed to enable individuals to discover the limits of their knowledge and how performance might be improved without referencing their ability to some norm. Robert Bjork (1999), along with many colleagues (e.g., Schmidt 1991), has put forward the notion that learning takes place predominantly through making mistakes, and that as a result, our task as educators or regulatory authorities is to construct situations that force individuals to encounter the limits of their ability. Termed "desirable difficulties," this concept is particularly important, as illustrated by Koriat et al. (2004), who have demonstrated that when we are given mistake-inducing tasks that may make us feel less comfortable/confident, we often show greater rates of retention and knowledge transfer than when left to our own devices because we often misjudge the extent to which we are learning (see Boehler et al. 2006; Eva 2009).

Test-enhanced learning offers one example of a strategy for inducing desirable difficulties as a pedagogical intervention, awareness of which is quickly spreading throughout the health professions education community (see Eva 2007; Kromann, Jensen, and Ringsted 2009; Larsen, Butler, and Roediger 2008). "Test-enhanced learning" describes enhanced learning that results from taking a test on to-be-learned material relative to spending the same amount of time restudying that material multiple times. In at least one study, the benefit of taking a test on learning was maintained for six months (Kromann et al. 2010). Greater awareness of this benefit may help inform the efforts of professional development facilitators by leading them to more deliberately deliver formative testing opportunities, thus encouraging greater participation on the part of learners in reviewing and improving their practice through well-constructed self-directed "assessment" activities, such as structured record audits and routine formative examinations.

Greater awareness of the value of desirable difficulties could also extend individuals' motivation to engage in the habit of self-directed assessment seeking (looking for opportunities to formally test themselves rather than relying on self-perceptions). In fact, while experiencing desirable difficulties has been argued to directly improve the learner's capacity to recall information by increasing the strength of the memory for the material, we have recently found that tests may also enhance learning by altering test takers' tendencies to seek out information of relevance to improving their performance. In a series of studies on self-monitoring (i.e., awareness of one's likelihood of answering correctly in the moment of being presented with a problem) undergraduate psychology students (Eva and Regehr 2007, 2011) and medical students (Agrawal, Norman, and Eva 2012) were asked to sit for sixty-item computer-based tests of general or medical knowledge, respectively. After completing the test students were four times as likely to search for information relevant to questions that they had to defer answering during the test (due to lack of confidence in their ability to answer the question correctly) relative to questions they chose to answer on the first opportunity (Eva and Regehr 2011). Similarly, they were twice as likely to search for information relevant to test questions if they had to deliberate extensively (>20 seconds) about whether they knew the answer relative to when they could decide quickly (<3 seconds) to answer or defer. Agrawal, Norman, and Eva found that the amount of time spent reviewing answers to individual questions was greater for questions medical students answered incorrectly relative to questions they answered correctly (even though feedback on their personal accuracy was not delivered explicitly). Perhaps more interestingly, however, was that within each of these categories, students were seen to spend more time reviewing questions in which the outcome was discordant with their expectations, spending the most time reviewing questions they answered incorrectly after indicating confidence in their response.

Taken as a whole, the material reviewed in this section generally points to a need to recognize that the recipient is a much more important component of the feedback process than the feedback intervention literature suggests. The recipient's perceptions of their own performance, the congruence between those perceptions and the feedback received, and the recipient's perceptions of the credibility and intent of the source of feedback will all influence the reception of that feedback and, in turn, influence the likelihood of engaging genuine effort toward performance improvement. In fact, we would go so far as to say that at a fundamental level, the recipient is the deciding factor in whether or not change occurs. We are led to this conclusion in part by very recent work indicating that inducing people to think about how others can help them achieve their goals can undermine individuals' motivations and thus make it less likely that those goals will be achieved. In a series of studies Fitzsimmons and Finkel (2011) report on the impact of "outsourcing" self-regulation. While they note that social support can benefit individuals in their pursuit of goals (Rusbult, Finkel, and Kumashiro 2009), they found that participants who were encouraged to think about how their partners could help them achieve health or academic goals were more likely to procrastinate and less likely to demonstrate behavior that would help them achieve those goals over the course of the following week relative to control groups of participants.

The change we hope to induce at the community level, therefore, is not one of eliminating the encouragement of self-directed learning. Rather the change we hope to induce is one of greater awareness that best practice in this area is not defined by the accuracy of one's self-assessment, that accurate self-assessment is not the mechanism whereby performance is improved, and that we should not judge the effectiveness of educational interventions solely by reliance on the perceptions of the learners. Instead, we should alter our models of self-directed learning to focus on encouraging self-directed assessment seeking. Doing so will involve shifting the conversation around the role of self-assessment toward the idea that the most important teaching we can do with respect to nurturing "good self-assessors" is to help learners recognize with humility that we are not uniquely privileged in understanding the strengths and limits of our own behaviors. Models of continuing professional development should, therefore, focus on creating opportunities for individuals to discover ways in which their performance can improve without prioritizing accuracy of self-assessment as the mechanism through which such improvements take place.

Conclusions

> Irony is a disciplinarian, feared only by those who do not know it, but cherished by those who do.
>
> Kierkegaard, *The Concept of Irony*

Continuing our appreciation of irony, throughout this chapter we have argued that we cannot trust self-assessment but should encourage it; that we need to influence self-assessment but should not change it; and that we can best improve the accuracy of self-assessment by ignoring it. We appreciate that these are difficult concepts, but the practical implication is that self-assessment does have a major role to play in performance improvement so long as it is *not* treated as the mechanism through which performance improves. When self-assessment is made the focus of individuals' determinations of what activities should be engaged to yield improved performance, it acts as a powerful lens through which all data and feedback are interpreted. All the research we can find suggests that the result of these processes is an interference with practice improvement, not its enhancement. Indeed, our judgments about ourselves drive as much as they reflect performance, but in ways that do not always appear rational. Helping poorer performers better understand that they lie in the lower quartile of their cohort is likely to be counterproductive. Such an understanding does not encourage them to improve, but rather discourages them from even trying. Thus the path to improving practice likely does not lie in helping people improve their self-assessment ability. Rather, it is more likely to lie in focusing instead on creating desirable difficulties that enable individuals to struggle effectively with their performance, prompting them to make mistakes from which they can learn. Ironically, such a process will also lead to the appearance of improved self-assessment by raising performance to meet our optimism rather than improving our actual self-assessment. Better that, however, than diminishing our optimism to the point that performance will not be raised. We are blinded by the insights provided through our self-assessment, but that is something to be taken advantage of, rather than something to be overcome.

THE COMPETENT MIND

Beyond Cognition

Annie S. O. Leung, Ronald M. Epstein,
and Carol-Anne E. Moulton

Judgment and decision making in the health care setting has mostly been conceptualized and researched as an individual activity—situated in the heads of physicians or health care professionals. Measurement of competence in medicine is therefore often a test of individual competence. Is this surgeon competent to perform the operations on her own? Can this nurse detect a patient who has become critically ill? Inarguably, there are essential competencies that need to be taught, learned, and assessed prior to stamping the seal of independence on any health care practitioner. This conceptualization of competence as an individual activity situated in the heads of practitioners is in part a product of the dominant discourse of cognitive psychology in health professional education over several decades. Yet the limitations of this model are obvious when we look at how health care is carried out on a daily basis. Practitioners are not working and making decisions in a vacuum. There is something more to competence than what is in the heads of individuals—their knowledge base, their skills, their judgment, and their decision-making abilities. Health care professionals draw conclusions from data collected from their environment. They are influenced by factors in their environment—some they are aware of and others they aren't. Recognition of this has led to a much greater emphasis on "teamwork" and "interprofessional care" in educational settings (Barr 1998; Reeves et al. 2008). Yet despite the obvious benefits of understanding the dynamics of how "teams" function in these contexts, some professionals struggle with the notion that they work within a team as many of their activities are individualized and lack constancy or stability that the construct of "team" implies.

We propose a model of competency that starts with an understanding of human individual cognition using a cognitive psychology framework, with the more recent considerations of the role of affect and intuition in cognitive functioning (Gigerenzer 2007; Lloyd and Reyna 2009; Peters et al. 2007; Reyna and Lloyd 2006). Through training, individuals gain experience and develop expertise within their field of study. This leads to the development of automaticity and freeing up of cognitive resources that can then be used for engaging in self-monitoring during everyday work; in other words, it leads to the ability to engage in mindful practice (Epstein 1999). The concept of mindful practice requires an understanding of not only the task-specific items of professional care but also the sociocultural influences on the individual and how that individual functions and contributes to health care in the setting of the larger health care team. After considering the individual components, we consider social elements of competence that may be embedded in coherent teams that have a long history and an established way of working together, or looser connections among members of "communities of care." Rather than viewing the cognitive and social models of competency separately, we will argue they are interdependent—that is, individuals generally cannot act competently unless supported in some way by a social structure, and teams cannot function without individuals who possess a minimal level of competence. Thus these two models need to be woven together and understood as one—the "shared mind." Through an understanding of the "shared mind" in the health care setting we can come closer to achieving excellence in health care.

The Competent Mind

Individual practitioners bring with them an accumulation of knowledge and skills in their particular area of expertise. In their uncertain and dynamic environment, they are required to pay attention to the pertinent cues around them that will require a change in plan, a call for help, or a different strategy. These cues come from several sources, contributing to the complexity of clinical practice; the patient or relative mentions the desire to give up, the patient anatomy in the operative field is not quite as it should be, the blood result is abnormal. What is known about cognition in this type of dynamic, uncertain environment? Through an exploration of the psychological, sociological, and human factors literatures, in this section we focus on the individual and explore several questions pertaining to individual cognition and expertise within the health care setting.

Cognitive Psychology of Attention

To understand how the expert thinks, it is useful to understand the ways in which cognitive psychologists have described human thinking based on years of experimental research of human attention.

Attention and Its Allocation   A basic premise in cognitive psychology is that human attention available for mental activity is limited (Cowan et al. 2005; Kahneman 1973; Moray 1967). In other words, many believe we have limited "space" for attentional resources, and once that threshold is reached, the mind tends to take mental shortcuts (i.e., heuristics) and oversimplify at the cost of accuracy (Kahneman, Slovic, and Tversky 1982). Different activities place different levels of demand on these resources: easy tasks require little attention and difficult tasks use up more attention. There is freedom within this model to be engaged attentively in several tasks simultaneously—to multitask, that is. Once our attentional threshold is reached, however, we are unable to attend to additional tasks without sacrificing attention to existing tasks. There are numerous environmental and task-related stimuli that are in essence competing for our attention at any given time. By definition, then, humans limit what they attend to and how attention is allocated at any given moment in time.

Two mechanisms have been have described concerning how individuals direct their attention: bottom-up and top-down (Connor, Egeth, and Yantis 2004). Bottom-up mechanisms operate on raw sensory input, rapidly and involuntarily shifting attention to salient visual features of potential importance, which has also been called the rule of involuntary attention (Remington, Johnston, and Yantis 1992). Some examples of these are hardwired

(Barcelo et al. 2006), such as bright lights, loud noises, or an artery "spurting" across the operating room that "steal" our attention, whereas others are acquired by association over time, such as our name being mentioned in a peripheral conversation (e.g., the cocktail party effect) (Corbetta and Shulman 2002; Neisser 1976). Top-down mechanisms implement our longer-term cognitive strategies, biasing attention. For example, the value the cue or stimulus holds for the individual may bias attention. One may never have noticed green Volkswagens prior to purchasing one; following a purchase they suddenly become much more "common." This is otherwise known as the "priming" effect in the psychology literature (LeBlanc, Norman, and Brooks 2001; Moray 1959; Simons 2000; Treisman 2006); once individuals are primed to anticipate a stimulus or cue, they are much more likely to pay attention to it when it occurs. In one such study, when participants were told to pay attention to voices in their right ear, they were more likely to notice voices in their right ear than similar voices in their left ear (Kahneman 1973). Through anticipation we are more likely to pay attention to the pertinent cues in the environment.

Situation Awareness   Building on the attention literature, with its theoretical and conceptual frameworks, is the theory of situation awareness found in the human factors literature and grounded in the measurement of human performance within complex, real-world situations. How do individuals use the information once it is perceived? How do they explain their environment? How do they predict what might happen next? Situation awareness most simply defined is a "constantly evolving picture of the state of the environment" (Jones and Endsley 1996). Several of the dominant models of situation awareness have their roots in early cognitive information processing models, which presume a linear progression of information processing from data collection to data integration to interpretation and prediction. Jones and Endsley's framework, for example, divides situation awareness into three levels: (1) perception of elements in the environment, (2) comprehension and integration of those elements into a coherent picture of the situation, and (3) projection of future states of the situation (ibid.). It is through a process of attaining and maintaining situation awareness that individual practitioners recognize subtle nuances or cues that don't quite fit, leading to a state of information gathering, decision making, and/or action.

Endsley (1995, 45) suggests "people are not helpless recipients of data from the environment but are active seekers of data in light of their goals." In the context of attention allocation, attending to important stimuli from the environment—that is, bottom-up processing—or actively seeking out new stimuli driven by operational goals—top-down processing—are synergistically working in parallel to enable the practitioner to obtain situation awareness (Beagan 2000; Casson 1983; Folk and Remington 2006; Higgins 1998). Psychophysical (Theeuwes 1992) and neurophysiological (Ogawa and Komatsu 2004) experiments in visual attention support the idea that bottom-up attention rapidly alerts us to salient items in our environment, but top-down attention modulates bottom-up signals with subsequent operations on sensory input by high-level cortex (Kim and Cave 1999; Lamy, Tsal, and Egeth 2003).

Systems of Thinking   Related to the theories of attention, Kahneman's work described two systems of thinking that people are engaged in through the course of their daily activities: system 1 (sometimes referred to as "automatic," intuitive, effortless, nonanalytic) and system 2 (sometimes referred to as "effortful," analytic, creative, deliberative) (Kahneman 1973). Automatic thought processes are evident when we are driving a familiar route and stop at a known stop sign. Effortful thought processes can be evoked when trying to drive to a new destination and there is a choice of routes, some of which may be superior at different times of day and may depend on road construction schedules. Choosing the best route requires deliberation and effort. In the context of clinical decision making, system 1 and system 2 have been viewed as being based on tacit and explicit knowledge respectively. Tacit knowledge are the skills, values, and experiences learned during observation and practice that are not explicitly stated or known to practitioners, whereas explicit knowledge is the conscious application of defined rules and objectively verifiable data to the patient's problem, such as evidence-based guidelines (Feinstein 1994; Goldman 1990; Polanyi 2003).

While this bimodal description of thought processes may be an oversimplification, and clinical decision making likely exists as a continuum where individuals operate in between these two extremes, it is nonetheless a useful way of considering the spectrum of attention required as experts perform different tasks that require varying amounts of effort. The attentional and thought-processing mechanisms we have described are similar in that they both lie along the spectrum between automatic (bottom-up and system 1) and effortful (top-down and system 2). A practitioner may use any combination and degree of these attentional and thought-processing mechanisms in any given moment of practice.

Cognitive Attention and Competence

Several theories on expert performance have built on these cognitive psychology principles for the purposes of trying to understand how experts utilize their limited cognitive capacity effectively. With the support of these theories on expertise, we will argue that how experts select and utilize cognitive mechanisms along the automatic-effortful spectrum is a basis for competency. We will also aim to clarify the meaning of the terms *experience, expertise*, and *expert* in the context of competency.

Competence as Automatic   According to models based in automaticity, individuals move from system 2 (requiring attention, effortful) to system 1 (automatic, intuitive) as they acquire experience. An experienced nurse taking a patient's blood pressure simply and effortlessly puts the cuff around the arm and takes the blood pressure while talking with the patient simultaneously, a task that would have required much more of her attention years before. As we become experienced in an activity, whether it is a physical task such as surgical knot tying or a mental task such as the diagnosis of a skin rash, the effort that is required to perform that task diminishes. The expert simply knows what to do and how to do it (Dreyfus, Athanasiou, and Dreyfus 1986). This function of automaticity is accomplished through the accumulation of many automatic resources, such as cognitive scripts, schemata, and pattern recognition, enabling the expert to engage in a quick, effortless, and automatic mode of functioning (Kahneman, Slovic, and Tversky 1982). Features of individual cases are no longer considered independently but form an overall pattern that is recognized effortlessly from years of experience and practice (Dreyfus, Athanasiou, and Dreyfus 1986). A neurologist may recognize Parkinson's disease within moments of meeting a patient, before professing the objective and subjective data to support it. A patient with upper quadrant pain, jaundice, and fever may "automatically" be recognized as having cholangitis.

As Dreyfus, Athanasiou, and Dreyfus (1986, 30) describe, "When things are proceeding normally, experts don't solve problems and don't make decisions: they do what normally works." While they state that interpretation plays a significant part in expert judgment, they view judgment predominantly as nonconscious and automatic. Their model celebrates the non-analytic nature of human expertise and focuses almost exclusively on the automatic mode of processing that experts are "normally" using, even in the unstructured problem areas. What is less clear in their model is what happens when things are not proceeding normally. What does expertise look like, for example, in the ill-defined or nonroutine areas of care? It is likely that system 1, the automatic mode, would be insufficient to deal with such issues in practice, and transitioning to a more effortful mode, or system 2, would be necessary.

This last point highlights our key argument in understanding how experts think in practice: expertise defined by automaticity does not equate to competency. Many errors committed by experienced clinicians are due to overreliance on their automatic mode (Regenbogen et al. 2007). In one of our studies with experienced surgeons (Moulton et al. 2010a), overreliance on the automatic mode was termed *drifting*. Surgeons described errors they made during the routine, "easy," or "boring" parts of the procedure where they felt they had "drifted" off the end of an acceptable acuity or attention spectrum. "It's the routine cases," one surgeon said. "Bile duct injuries always happen in easy gall bladders, right? That's what happened here. It was an easy case. We were chatting and obviously not being as diligent as we should have been" (Moulton et al. 2010a, 1575). Thus, conceptualizing expertise exclusively as the accrual and efficient use of nonanalytic resources and load-reducing automatic processes is likely insufficient (Eva 2002).

Competence as Effortful   Contrary to the Dreyfus, Athanasiou, and Dreyfus model of expertise as primarily a celebration of automaticity, Bereiter and Scardamalia's *Surpassing Ourselves* (1993) offers a model that stresses the importance of effort, with emphasis placed on management of the ill-defined and unstructured areas of practice. While they acknowledge automaticity in expertise, they focus on the effortful mode of thinking through their distinction between an experienced nonexpert, who relies on routine and automatic thinking, and the true expert, who explicitly sets out to identify the subtle complexities of situations. By addressing and read-dressing the problems of daily practice through an effortful process, true experts develop a deep understanding of the particular systems they are working with. Thus expertise in their model is achieved when one constantly and intentionally engages with one's environment during the routines of daily practice.

Similar to the idea of an experienced expert, Bransford, in his book *How People Learn* (2000), describes an adaptive expert as one who is able to efficiently solve previously encountered tasks and generate new procedures for new tasks (Hatano and Inagaki 1986). Contrast two types of Japanese sushi experts as an example—one excels at following a fixed recipe and the other prepares sushi differently each time depending on context, such as the nature of today's raw ingredients, the preferences of the consumer, and perhaps even the time of year. These appear to represent two very different types of expertise, one that is relatively routinized and one that is flexible and more adaptable to external demands. Similarly, experts have been characterized as either "merely skilled" or "highly competent," and more colorfully as either "artisans" or "virtuosos" (Miller 1978). Adaptability allows experts to recognize when highly practiced rules and principles do not apply in certain situations, where others, in the same situations, typically attempt to use a previously learned procedure (Bereiter and Scardamalia 1993; Gott et al. 1992). But how much of this matching of appropriate cognitive activity to a particular task is intentional? How much control do we have over it? How do experts ensure they pay attention to the pertinent cues when required, and what does this recruitment of additional cognitive resources look like?

Competence as "Slowing Down When You Should"   This transitioning between the automatic mode and the effortful mode in practice has been a focus of study in the surgical literature and provides some insight into what this transition looks like, what factors initiate it, and how it is experienced by surgeons in their operative practice (Moulton et al. 2007; Moulton et al. 2010a, 2010b). Transitioning from the automatic mode to the effortful mode was referred to as "slowing down when you should" and described the cognitive refocusing or increased attention directed toward a particular task during the critical moments of practice. Although this phenomenon was explored in the surgical setting, we and others have suggested its applicability in other complex health care environments (Ajjawi and Smith 2010; Samuels and Fetzer 2009; Varpio, Schryer, and Lingard 2009), and thus we describe it in detail here.

Surgeons described two types of slowing down moments: *proactively planned* moments during the procedure that had been anticipated by the surgeon preoperatively and *situationally responsive* moments when unexpected "cues" or stimuli alerted the surgeon to the unanticipated need to pay more attention (Moulton et al. 2010b). Outside of medicine the same slowing down moments may be experienced by drivers as they approach a known dangerous intersection on a regular route home each day (i.e., proactively planned) or swerve to avoid a collision with a pedestrian who has run out in front of the car (i.e., situationally responsive). Proactively planned and situationally responsive moments may share a similar cognitive basis as top-down and bottom-up attentional mechanisms respectively, as described previously.

Four manifestations of the slowing down phenomenon were observed in the operating room (Moulton et al. 2010a). The most extreme manifestation was described as "stopping," when surgeons stopped operating to pause or regroup for the purposes of gathering new information or to make sure they were on the right track. Second, surgeons were sometimes observed "removing distractions" when confronted by the critical or unexpected moments, asking for conversations to be taken outside or for music to be turned off. At times, surgeons appeared to simply "focus more intently" on the task at hand, removing themselves from conversations but allowing them to continue on around them. Finally, surgeons were observed to engage in what appeared to be "fine-tuning" activities where the surgeon focused on the task momentarily when necessary for the purposes of staying on course and out of trouble. This concept of fine-tuning appears to be in contradistinction to the concept of "drifting" described in the sections above, where surgeons found themselves in trouble as they lost focus during the routine aspects of care. Fine-tuning activities seemed to be micro slow down moments— perhaps thousands occur in a single operation—where surgeons purposefully exerted attention to ensure they stayed on track. This comparison between drifting and fine-tuning led to the conceptualization of "inattentive" and "attentive" automaticity, respectively (Moulton et al. 2010a).

In contrast to the Dreyfus, Athanasiou, and Dreyfus model (1986) that celebrates the automatic functioning of the expert as largely effortless, our observations suggest that within automaticity, expert surgeons maintain a level of attention over and above the necessary level that would be expected for "automatic" functioning (Moulton et al. 2010a)—even during the most routine portions of their work. These surgeons—consciously or unconsciously—remained focused and attentive, reinvesting the freed-up cognitive resources afforded them through their development of expertise back into monitoring activities of the case. In their interviews, they described a state of "heightened awareness" or vigilance especially during the routine cases to ensure they did not "drift" into trouble. In the surgeons' view, "drifting" was a negative by-product of automaticity, a state of inattention that made them more vulnerable to error. Given these two descriptions of "automaticity," we proposed that being in an automatic mode was not an "all or none" phenomenon, but rather could be further characterized by how much attention is reinvested back into monitoring activities during the case.

"Slowing down when you should" can then be viewed as a competency that differentiates the experienced nonexpert or nonadaptive expert from a true adaptive expert. With this distinction between expertise and competency based on individual cognitive mechanisms, recent research focuses on strategies individuals can use to become a "competent expert."

The Mindful Competent Mind

Metacognition

We have thus far focused our discussion of individual competency from the perspective of cognition, which according to Neisser (1976, 1) is "the activity of knowing: the acquisition, organization, and use of knowledge." Practitioners, however, because they are in a dynamic and complex environment, are required to maintain some degree of awareness not only of the external situation (e.g., the operating field, the clinical encounter) but also of their interior landscape (e.g., whether they are feeling anxious, whether the situation is aversive to them). This form of conscious self-awareness is called *metacognition*, which is defined as "one's knowledge concerning one's own cognitive processes and products or anything related to them" (Flavell 1976, 232). In other words, metacognition is the regulation of cognition, or "thinking about thinking" (Flavell 1979). Other terms to describe this internal regulatory process are *reflective intelligence*, "the ability to make one's own mental processes the object of conscious observation (Skemp 1979, 175), and *self-monitoring*, "an ability to attend, moment to moment, to our own actions; curiosity to examine the effects of those actions; and willingness to use those observations to improve behavior and patterns of thinking in the future" (Epstein, Siegel, and Silberman 2008, 5).

Paying attention to both the external situation and internal landscape requires effort and takes up cognitive resources (Kahneman 1973). Cognitive capacity and cognitive load is an area of research that encompasses much more than attention and is beyond the scope of this chapter (Plass, Moreno, and Brünken 2010). However, a crude simplification would be to view mental resources as shared between cognitive and metacognitive processes, with cognitive processes taking priority. In this view, a "competent expert" in routine situations has residual cognitive capacity to reinvest into metacognitive processes and "fine-tune" their performance. With our expanding view of competence beyond the "competence as cognition" model, the importance of metacognitive monitoring in health professionals has been recognized in various research programs in medical education (Epstein, Siegel, and Silberman 2008; Eva and Regehr 2005; Regehr and Eva 2006).

Metacognition and Automaticity

Monitoring cognitive processes and activities assumes that we have access to them and have some control over them. In unfamiliar situations where effortful analytic problem solving is required, our cognitive processes are explicit (e.g., what are my options and what are the pros and cons of each?). In contrast, automatic functioning using tacit knowledge by definition takes place without effort through processes that are thought to be beyond our control (e.g., expert surgeons may find it difficult to describe the discrete hand positions involved in knot tying) (Eva and Norman 2005; Nisbett and Wilson 1977). From this perspective, explicit cognitive processes may be easily monitored (e.g., are there options I haven't thought of?), but automatic or tacit cognitive processes may more easily evade metacognitive monitoring. Some have suggested that the "drifting" described in the slowing down phenomenon is beyond the control of the subject working in such routine or "automatic" conditions—referred to as "involuntary automaticity"—with the argument that this could be a valid medico-legal defense in the court of law (Toft and Gooderham 2009).

However, as we noted in the "slowing down" study, the surgeons' ability to attend to their environment on a moment-by-moment basis was to some degree determined by conscious decisions about how they would re-invest freed-up cognitive resources. Some chose to engage in peripheral, extraneous conversations, running the risk of "drifting," while others chose to purposefully monitor their situation and engage in "fine-tuning." The spectrum from inattentive to attentive automaticity points to the importance of the metacognitive monitoring process to "pay attention" not only to the moment of practice but also to our own thoughts, feelings, and intuitive forces (Garofalo 1986). Thus "attentive automaticity" challenges the notion that automatic processes that utilize tacit knowledge are inaccessible; rather, these automatic processes that exist "outside of everyday cognitive awareness" may be awakened, accessed, and monitored with effort and practice.

Manifestations of Attentive Automaticity

Before we can monitor these tacit cognitive processes through metacognitive awareness, what tacit cognitive processes look like in practice and where they come from should be understood. *Subsidiary awareness, gut feeling*, and *intuition* are all terms that have been used to describe the tacit knowledge that experts possess and cognitive processes that follow. The ability of practitioners to recognize when situations are aberrant and require more attention and focus or when a patient is "not quite right" has been described as a level of "subsidiary awareness" (Epstein 1999; Polanyi 2003). Subsidiary awareness makes accessible the flow of unprocessed experience (Polanyi 2003) through a preattentive phase (Austin 1999), where the brain rapidly scans a wide array of perceptions, detects conspicuous features, and relegates some information to the background, all before the content of the perception that forms the objective data of a clinical case is analyzed. Gigerenzer, in his book *Gut Feelings: The Intelligence of the Unconscious* (2007), reminds us that simple cognitive heuristics (i.e., mental shortcuts) are essential for accurate and quick choices and suggests they be celebrated for their role in our successes. This concept of automaticity is central to Reyna and Lloyd's "fuzzy-trace" theory (2006), where their work in the medical field has demonstrated that expert clinicians use less information than we might expect when making decisions and judgments, relying instead on their "gut feelings," or as they describe, the "gist" of the situation. Klein, the founder of the naturalistic decision making movement, suggests this intelligence of the unconscious is in fact key to survival in many life-threatening workplace situations. He describes firefighters evacuating buildings intuitively only to realize subsequently that the sensation of heat underneath their feet unconsciously alerted them to the impending floor collapse (Klein 1999).

It has been hypothesized that intuition comes from emotions and sensory experiences that are packaged with our learning experiences and knowledge and form part of our memory; when the memory is retrieved, the emotions and sensory experiences are automatically retrieved—often influencing behavior and decision making (Damasio 1999; Schmidt, Norman, and Boshuizen 1990). McNaughton and LeBlanc (chapter 3) provide an in-depth review of the neuroscience and cognitive literature challenging the historical separation of thinking and feeling, a paradigm that has largely been replaced by the prevailing view that cognitive and emotional processes are integral to each other and operate in parallel. Damasio's "somatic marker" hypothesis proposes that, rather than being the antithesis of reasoning, emotions are indispensable to decision making (Damasio 1999). Thus clinical judgment is based on an interdependence of action, cognition, memory, and emotion (Damasio 1994).

Habits of Mindful Practice

Mindfulness has been described as a key strategy for harnessing metacognition to monitor automatic or intuitive processes and for achieving a state of "attentive automaticity." Rather than being viewed as an exercise in meditation, which many people perceive as a practice that "empties the mind," mindful practice is "conscious and intentional attentiveness to the present situation—the raw sensations, thoughts, and emotions as well as the interpretations, judgments, and heuristics that one applies to a particular situation" (Epstein, Siegel, and Silberman 2008, 9). The awareness that comes with mindful practice appears to stabilize our attention and make the contents of the mind more available for understanding (Germer, Siegel, and Fulton 2005; Kabat-Zinn 2005). It helps us avoid going on "automatic pilot"—and thus helps us become more reflective and more flexible in our responses (Bargh and Chartrand 1999). As expertise provides cognitive space, practitioners can choose how they reinvest their freed-up cognitive resources. Adopting a stance of mindfulness through the habits of mindful practice is a conscious decision that we believe is essential for the competent mind.

Habits that can be developed to improve our ability to be mindful during our clinical activities include attentive observation, critical curiosity, beginner's mind, and presence (Epstein, Siegel, and Silberman 2008; Moulton and Epstein 2011). Attentive observation includes vigilance and openness to the unexpected, in details pertaining to both the external world (e.g., abnormal heart sounds, aberrant blood values) and ourselves (e.g., our perception and responses to cues in our environment and to our emotions). Critical curiosity, or "seeing the world as it is and not as we would like it to be" (Epstein 2003a, 7), is the practice of tolerating and welcoming doubt and uncertainty into practice. Rather than withdrawing from emotionally or cognitively difficult situations (e.g., an angry patient, a surgical mishap) or blaming the situation on others, the physician can approach the situation with openness: "How did this come to be? Are there factors that I haven't considered?" The adoption of a beginner's mind—to see a situation freshly, with a willingness to set aside assumptions that have previously been made—is a healthy state that allows for "contradictory ideas to be held simultaneously" and for new ideas to emerge. For a practitioner, this could mean that a rule invites an exception, that the diagnosis needs revisiting, or that the tumor she thought was resectable is not. Observations are considered conditional (Langer 1997). The certainty of knowing for a fact is replaced with the willingness to look for possibilities and prepare for the unexpected, recognizing that all conflicts and dilemmas do not need to be reconciled immediately. The habit of presence means avoiding preoccupation and distraction and being "in the moment." Cognitive resources are invested back into the situation. When such a state is achieved, clinicians may be more likely to appropriately "respond" to the slowing down moments, focusing and remaining purposeful in a productive manner—rather than missing the cue altogether or inappropriately "reacting" with unproductive anxiety (Asher and Epstein 2005). Engaging in the state of mindful practice assists us in our efforts to seek, integrate, and respond to both "external" and "internal" data about our own performance (Epstein, Siegel, and Silberman 2008). This state of mindful practice is linked to the ability to adequately engage in the process of self-monitoring in practice.

Researchers propose that mindful awareness can be developed that will disentangle set pathways of automatic responses, engaging some activities and disengaging others so that information flow is altered. This ability to attend to the most important information while inhibiting irrelevant information has been described as *executive attention*. In other words, executive attention allows mental representations derived from memory and present goals to be maintained in a highly active state in the face of distraction (Conway et al. 2005). The attentional control achieved helps us recognize when we are distracted, fatigued, or biased and may help to recalibrate the alerting, orienting, or executive function, which has been proposed to offer benefits of personal well-being and professional practice (Epstein, Siegel, and Silberman 2008; Siegel 2007). Results of recent studies suggest that mindfulness can be learned even by experienced practitioners, and that subjective difference in physicians' practices (which often correlate with observational measures) can result (Krasner et al. 2009). Further evidence from functional magnetic resonance imaging has demonstrated focal increases in cortical thickness (Lazar et al. 2005) and changes in neural pathways that accompany intensive mindfulness training (Farb et al. 2007); these changes correlate to areas of the brain that regulate sensory input, executive function, and emotions. Furthermore, it has been suggested that intentionally creating an effortful state of awareness will lead to synaptic growth where effortful states become effortless traits of mindfulness in an individual over time (Epstein, Siegel, and Silberman 2008). This phenomenon of effortlessness—when a person's full engagement in an activity provides ongoing impetus for attention and action—has been described as an autotelic experience commonly known as "flow" (Csikszentmihalyi and Csikszentmihalyi 2000).

The Competent Mindful Mind in Context

With a foundational knowledge of the cognitive and metacognitive underpinnings of individual competence and expertise, it is important to bring these mechanisms that reside in the individual into the real-world context and to consider the situational and cultural factors that can impact judgment and decision making in practice. The dynamic and complex environment of clinical practice brings with it various contextual factors that influence practitioners' ability to be mindful. The ability to maintain awareness of both the external environment and the internal landscape in face of these contextual factors can be described as *situated competence—* competency that is necessarily contextual (Klass 2007).

Situational Competency and Cognition

In any moment of clinical practice there are numerous competing priorities that practitioners must actively balance—trainees to teach, grant applications to write, meetings to attend. Hospital administrators want efficiency. In-hospital patients need attention. Several factors have been identified that influence surgeons' ability to "slow down" appropriately. Fatigue, for example, diminishes an individual's ability to remain attentive and focused (Kahneman 1973). One surgeon acknowledged that, "My decision making and judgment when I was tired or frustrated at one or two in the morning was not as crisp" (Moulton et al. 2010b, 1024). Distractions are also a part of practice that may affect the practitioner's ability to slow down (Hsu et al. 2008). As one surgeon described, "I may … ask for quiet in the room or to reduce distractions, that sort of thing" (Moulton et al. 2010b, 1021). With our understanding of the limited attentional capacity, these responsibilities and factors place pressures on the practitioner in their attempt to direct their attention to the patient in front of them. Thus there is a real-world tension between the fundamental need to do "what is best" for the patient in front of the practitioner and the multiple other responsibilities and expectations that practitioners must fulfill (Leung et al. 2011). Some of these pressures have been acknowledged in research pertaining to practitioner burnout (Krasner et al. 2009; Shanafelt et al. 2010) and may be discussed at morbidity and mortality rounds within hospitals as causes of error requiring a systems-based solution (Orlander, Barber, and Fincke 2002). Beyond what is acknowledged and discussed, however, the sociocultural milieu with its various social pressures may be an even more powerful influence on cognition.

Social Identity and the Culture of Medicine

Practitioners make decisions and apply judgments not in isolation but within a powerful social and cultural context. Although the effect of these social forces is informal, unmentioned, and largely hidden (Hafferty 1991), it is not necessarily subtle and can influence practitioners' judgment and decision making. Studies demonstrating cultural differences in attention allocation support the notion that allocation of attention is highly malleable and subject to learned strategic adjustments (Meyer et al. 1995; Meyer and Kieras 1997a, 1997b; Rogoff et al. 1993). There is also increasing evidence that systems of thought exist in homeostasis with the social practices that surround them (Nisbett et al. 2001). In other words, social practices and cognitive processes could support or "prime" one another (Hong et al. 2000).

The concept of image management—the external social pressures in the moment to manage one's image and impression on others—as it relates to judgment has been explored in surgery (Jin et al., forthcoming). Actions and behaviors are determined by a combination of "what we think of ourselves" and "what we think others think of us" (Monrouxe 2010). The former, "who I think I am," is an internalized identity developed through group membership and the socialization process. The latter, "who I think you think I am," is relevant to external, in-the-moment social pressures to manage one's image and impression on others. Each will be elaborated below in turn.

Social identity is an aspect of an individual's self-concept that derives from the individual's membership in a group (Gergen and Davis 1985). A practitioner's professional identity, derived from belonging to the larger social group formed by health care practitioners, is constructed by a three-stage process involving adaptation to professional culture, internalization of professional identity, and demonstration of solidarity with other professionals (Dryburgh 1999). It is easier for an individual whose personal identities are consistent with the new professional role to take on the professional identity, and where there is incongruence between personal and professional identities, "identity dissonance" is created (Monrouxe 2010). The pressure to conform to mainstream expectations around behaviors, attitudes, and belief systems is well documented in health care trainees entering training programs as well as individuals who are not part of the mainstream (e.g., cultural/religious minorities, women in predominantly male environments) (Beagan 2001; Costello 2005; Monrouxe 2010).

The external pressures of "what others think of me" can be understood with Goffman's description of how individuals are "actors" playing roles in social situations. Image management involves learning to follow expected social scripts for behavior in different situations (Goffman 1959). For example, the surgical culture stresses certitude, decisiveness, and confidence (DelVecchio Good 1995). Thus a surgeon may feel the need to manifest these qualities in the operating room despite feelings of uncertainty, and may avoid calling for help. In the face of uncertainty, there likely exists a tension felt by the surgeon between needing to "appear" certain and actually "being" certain.

Sociocultural Context and Attentional Capacity

The implications of the situational pressures and the social pressures of image management are apparent when considered in the context of attentional capacity. As discussed previously, we have limited attentional capacity, and monitoring what is unfolding in any particular situation requires investment of energy and attention. To engage in these monitoring activities, then, requires some available capacity that in stressful or uncertain situations may not seem readily available. It has been shown that thoughts, feelings, and emotions during any given moment "eat up" a portion of an individual's attention, leaving less cognitive reserve or spare capacity available for other functions (Kahneman 1973). McNaughton and LeBlanc (chapter 3) discuss in great detail the influence of emotion on a range of cognitive functions (e.g., perception, attention, and decision making), as well as how cognitive functions can affect the emotional experience. The literature referenced by McNaughton and LeBlanc together with findings from our own study suggest that the ability to think clearly, to gather and process information in the moment of crisis, can be jeopardized by consuming thoughts and emotions associated with image management. As one surgeon in the "slowing down" study said, "My efforts during these moments of crises were consumed with the anxiety I was feeling...intermixed with feelings of inadequacy, uncertainty, reputation, and ego" (Moulton and Epstein 2011). Another surgeon described the social pressure of hospital hierarchy felt when operating with a more senior surgeon: "Even if it is my case...you let the person do something and you think, Gee, I hope we didn't do that...more out of respect for the surgeon, instead of respect for the patient" (Moulton et al. 2010b; Moulton and Epstein 2011). When cognitive resources are reaching their limit during these critical, unexpected, or uncertain "slowing down" moments, further consumption of resources by the internal and external pressures brought on by sociocultural forces may interfere with the thought processes, the monitoring activities, and the action execution of the task at hand. A surgeon thinking about his reputation while also disquieted by the anxiety of dealing with a surgical mishap may be experiencing cognitive load issues; as a result he may have, at that moment, a relative lack of resources to deal with the immediate event or anticipate future events.

Furthermore, the strength model of self-control states that acts of self-control (e.g., inhibiting thoughts, exaggerating emotional expressions) consume and deplete inner limited resources required for subsequent attention control (Schmeichel and Baumeister 2010). Thus, in ways similar to fatigue and distractions, sociocultural pressures may compete for the same attentional pool that practitioners depend on to maintain situation awareness. Evidence suggests that, with practice, self-control may become less effortful and that regular exercises in self-control help make effortless what was once an effortful act of control (Gailliot et al. 2007). Therefore, understanding sociocultural pressures (e.g., internal ego, external hierarchy) and their effects on cognition would empower the practitioner to further self-reflect and engage in "mindful practice." When we are able to free up our cognitive capacity from the anxieties of uncertainty, reputation, ego, and inadequacy, our limited resources can then be devoted to the challenges of the clinical situation at hand.

The Shared Mind

Health care practitioners work in the setting of health care teams, or "communities of practice," and depend on the environment and those around them to deliver excellent care. Recognized widely in the medical literature and beyond is the concept that knowledge and skill are shared among all members of a team or larger social unit, whether it is a team working in the operating room, a primary care physician's network of subspecialty consultants, or the nurses and medical assistants working in an outpatient office. Terms such as *distributed cognition* (Hutchins 1995), *collaborative cognition*

(Rogoff 1998), *distributed situation awareness* (Salmon 2009), *team situation awareness* (Salas et al. 1995; Wellens 1993), and *collective competence* (as described in chapter 2 of this volume) have all been used to capture the synergistic effect of a group of people sharing information and making decisions together while working toward a common goal. Our model of professional competency thus far has stressed the importance of understanding the individual situated in the health care setting, with an appreciation for the cognitive, the psychosocial, and the cultural components of competency in that setting. Yet individuals work in the setting of larger social units and this also needs to be integrated into the model of mindful practice, leading us to a newer term, *shared mind*. The concept of shared mind refers to the "ways in which new ideas and perspectives can emerge through the sharing of thoughts, feelings, perceptions, meanings and intentions among two or more people" (Epstein and Street 2011). At the foundation of the "shared mind" model lie the concepts of collaborative cognition, attunement, and sensemaking.

Collaborative cognition is the process of compensating for deficits in each others' ability to process information and solve problems, especially in high-stress high-stakes situations (Epstein and Street 2011; Meegan and Berg 2002). Clinicians engage in collaborative cognition in the form of team rounds in teaching hospitals, where often the group arrives at better decisions than any one individual. Similarly, in the operating room the surgeon can rely on others to process information and provide alternative options of care during stressful situations. While collaborative cognition refers to problem solving, the concept of *attunement* refers to a feeling of being on the "same wavelength," or "feeling in stride" with another person in various interpersonal interactions: patients and clinicians (Bálint 2000; Branch and Malik 1993; Meegan and Berg 2002; Suchman and Matthews 1988), supervisors and trainees (Branch et al. 2009; Palmer 2007), health care teams (Norton and Bowers 2001), and communities of care (Haidet et al. 2009; Wenger 1998). A neural basis of attunement based on functional neuroimaging studies has been proposed (Gallese, Keysers, and Rizzolatti 2004; Pfeifer and Dapretto 2009; Rizzolatti and Craighero 2004). Together, attunement and collaborative cognition contribute to *sensemaking* within a team or an organization, in which collective brainstorming and sharing experiences generate meaning (Kreps 2009; Weick 1995). Sensemaking is an iterative process where its products (e.g., shared meaning) can in turn influence subsequent understanding and decisions, thus allowing for expanded perspectives and consideration of values and preferences in complex situations. This process is applicable to both well-established and structured teams (e.g., a liver transplant team) as well as more loosely constructed communities of practice (e.g., a primary care physician's referral network) (Epstein 1999; Fioratou et al. 2010; Haidet et al. 2009; Wenger 1998). Although originally described in the context of patient-physician interactions, shared mind may also be relevant in clinician-clinician and supervisor-trainee interactions. With shared mind, the responsibility for attention may be distributed, curiosity arises through individual as well as dyadic interactions, flexibility refers to the generation and elaboration of a shared idea or emotion, and presence refers to the broader sphere of engagement among members of the group. Similar to how "mindfulness" in an individual enables metacognitive monitoring of cognitive content and processes to control attention, shared mindfulness, explored in aviation, is described as "a state of mindfulness achieved conjointly, whereby, in the communicative interaction, the individuals involved are in an active state of attending, responding, and perceiving information correctly. As a result, they are continually updating, attuned, and open to incoming data that are unexpected, disconfirming, improbable, implicit, and/or contested" (Krieger 2005, 138). Thus, qualities of mindful organizations and teams—as outlined by Weick and Sutcliffe—mirror those of individuals (Weick and Sutcliffe 2001). Parallel to how "mindfulness" is the foundation for appropriate transitioning in individual competency, "shared mindfulness" is the foundation for appropriate transitioning in shared models of competency and requires ongoing research in the health care setting.

Conclusion

Slowing down when you should is a term that describes a competency in switching between automatic and effortful modes of practice in planned and unplanned situations, while also avoiding inattentive automaticity (e.g., drifting, mindlessness, overconcreteness). In this chapter we have explored how this phenomenon manifests during clinical practice both as intrapsychic and interpersonal processes. We have hinted at, though have not directly explored, how the capacities of mindful practice can be cultivated.

At minimum, clinicians should learn the basics of human cognition to develop an awareness for when they are practicing at their best and when they are not. This capacity is especially important for clinician-educators, who can share that interoceptive self-knowledge with trainees—being "conspicuously mindful" (Epstein 2003b) on the one hand, and also, in a powerful gesture of humility and curiosity, being transparent when they are not (Dyche and Epstein 2011). Approaching mindfulness as a skill sets up the need for more understanding of mindfulness training in the health professions, which may include more formal activities, such as meditation, or more informal practices, such as taking "mindful moments" during the workday. These approaches have gained increasing acceptance not only in medicine but in other fields that require high-level cognition under stress (Lesser 2009; Weick, Sutcliffe, and Obstfeld 2005). Our view is that simply reflecting on one's actions outside of the clinic setting is insufficient. Rather, modeling (Epstein 2003b), use of reflective questions (Borrell-Carrio and Epstein 2004), and an institutional culture that promotes reflective practice are all necessary. Work employing multiformat approaches to cultivating interpersonal and intrapersonal mindfulness suggests that such an approach can enhance quality of care while also enhancing clinicians' quality of life (Krasner et al. 2009).

Our work points to a new model of competence that integrates individual and collective factors, acknowledging that cognition is to some degree shared across individuals. This more complete model of competence focuses on communities of practice and on individual expertise and, importantly, the interactions between them, recognizing that humans possess both individual wisdom and social connectedness. Future research should explore in greater depth the nature of this "situated shared competence."

REFERENCES

Accreditation Council for Graduate Medical Education (ACGME). 2011. 2001–present: Outcome project. http://www.acgme.org/Outcome (accessed December 3, 2011).

Accreditation Council for Graduate Medical Education: ACGME Outcomes Project. 2003a. Common program requirements: General competencies. http://www.acgme. org/outcome/comp/GeneralCompetenciesStandards21307.pdf (accessed March 3, 2010).

——. 2003b. Timeline-Working guidelines. http://www.acgme.org/outcome/project/ timeline/ TIMELINE_index_frame.htm (accessed February 10, 2010).

Adolphs, R., D. Tranel, and T. W. Buchanan. 2005. Amygdala damage impairs emotional memory for gist but not details of complex stimuli. *Nature Neuroscience* 8 (4): 512–518.

Agrawal, S., G. R. Norman, and K. W. Eva. 2012. Influences on students' self-regulated learning after test completion. *Medical Education* 46:326–335.

Ahmed, S. 2004. *The cultural politics of emotion.* New York: Routledge.

Ajjawi, R., and M. Smith. 2010. Clinical reasoning capability: Current understanding and implications for physiotherapy educators. *Focus on Health Professional Education: A Multi-Disciplinary Journal* 12 (1): 60–73.

Albanese, R. 1989. Competency-based management education. *Journal of Management Development* 8: 66–76.

Alloy, L. B., and L. Y. Abramson. 1979. Judgment of contingency in depressed and nondepressed students: Sadder but wiser? *Journal of Experimental Psychology: General* 108:441–485.

Amalberti, R., Y. Auroy, D. Berwick, and P. Barach. 2005. Five system barriers to achieving ultrasafe health care. *Annals of Internal Medicine* 142:756–764.

American Board of Medical Specialties (ABMS). 1999. MOC competencies and criteria. http://www.abms.org/Maintenance_of_Certification/MOC_competencies.aspx (accessed November 13, 2008).

American Medical Association (AMA). 2008. CPT Coding, billing and insurance. http://www.ama-assn.org/ama/pub/physician-resources/solutions-managing-your-practice/coding-billing-insurance/cpt.page (accessed November 24, 2011).

———. 2010a. AMA position statement: Competency-based training in medical education 2010. http://www.ama.com.au/node/4495 (accessed December 1, 2011).

———. 2010b. Initiative to transform medical education (ITME): The importance of assessing behavioral competencies in the medical school admissions process (accessed December 1, 2011).

Anema, M. G., and J. McCoy. 2010. *Competency-based nursing education: Guide to achieving outstanding learning outcomes.* New York: Springer.

Archer, J. 2010. State of the science in health professional education: Effective feedback. *Medical Education* 44:101–108.

Aristotle. 1961. *Poetics.* Trans. S. H. Butcher. New York: Hill and Wang.

Arora, S., R. Aggarwal, P. Moran, P. Sirimanna, A. Crochet, R. Darzi, R. Kneebone, and N. Sevdalis. 2011. Mental practice: Effective stress management training for novice surgeons. *Journal of the American College of Surgeons* 212 (2): 225–233.

Arora, S., N. Sevdalis, R. Aggarwal, P. Sirimanna, A. Darzi, and R. Kneebone. 2010. Stress impairs psychomotor performance in novice laparoscopic surgeons. *Surgical Endoscopy* 24 (10): 2588–2593.

Asher, B. F., and R. M. Epstein. 2005. Managing the stress of surgical complications. In *Complications in pediatric otolaryngology,* ed. G. Josephson and D. Wohl, 23–28. Boca Raton, FL: Taylor & Francis.

Association for Medical Education in Europe (AMEE). 2011. AMEE annual meeting programme. http://www.amee.org/documents/AMEE%202011%20Final%20Programme.pdf (accessed September 10, 2011).

Association of American Medical Colleges (AAMC). 2011. 2011 AAMC annual meeting thought leader sessions. https://www.aamc.org/meetings/2011_annual_meeting/255086/thoughtleaders.html (accessed September 10, 2011).

Association of American Medical Colleges-Howard Hughes Medical Institute Committee. 2009. Scientific foundations for future physicians. http://www.hhmi.org/grants/pdf/08–209_AAMC-HHMI_report.pdf (accessed December 8, 2011).

Association of Faculties of Medicine of Canada. 2010. Future of medical education in Canada (FMEC): A collective vision for MD education. http://www.afmc.ca/fmec/pdf/collective_vision.pdf (accessed July 5, 2011).

Austin, J. H. 1999. *Zen and the brain: Toward an understanding of meditation and consciousness.* Cambridge, MA: MIT Press.

Bálint, M. 2000. *The doctor, his patient and the illness.* 2nd ed. Edinburgh: Churchill Livingstone.

Barcelo, F., C. Escera, M. J. Corral, and J. A. Perianez. 2006. Task switching and novelty processing activate a common neural network for cognitive control. *Journal of Cognitive Neuroscience* 18 (10): 1734–1748.

Bargh, J. A., and T. L. Chartrand. 1999. The unbearable automaticity of being. *American Psychologist* 54:462–479.

Barr, H. 1998. Competent to collaborate: Towards a competency-based model for interprofessional education. *Journal of Interprofessional Care* 12 (2): 181–187.

Barzun, J. 1988. Multiple-choice flunks out. *New York Times.* October 11.

Beagan, B. L. 2000. Neutralizing differences: Producing neutral doctors for (almost) neutral patients. *Social Science & Medicine* 51 (8): 1253–1265.

———. 2001. "Even if I don't know what I'm doing I can make it look like I know what I'm doing": Becoming a doctor in the 1990s. *Canadian Review of Sociology* 38 (3): 275–292.

Bechara, A., A. R. Damasio, H. Damasio, and S. Anderson. 1994. Insensitivity to future consequences following damage to the prefrontal cortex. *Cognition* 50:7–15.

Bechara, A., D. Tranel, and H. Damasio. 2000. Characterization of the decision-making deficit in patients with ventromedial prefrontal cortex lesions. *Brain* 123:2189–2202.

Becker, F., and F. Steele. 1995. *Workplace by design: Mapping the high performance workscape.* San Francisco: Jossey-Bass.

Bereiter, C. 1995. A dispositional view of transfer. In *Teaching for transfer: Fostering generalization in learning,* ed. A. McKeough, J. Lupart, and A. Marini, 21–34. Mahwah, NJ: Erlbaum Associates.

———. 1997. Situated cognition and how to overcome it. In *Situated cognition: Social, semiotic, and psychological perspectives,* ed. D. Kirshner and J. A. Whitson, 281–300. Hillsdale, NJ: Erlbaum Associates.

———. 2002. *Education and mind in the knowledge age.* Mahwah, NJ: Lawrence Erlbaum Associates.

Bereiter, C., and M. Scardamalia. 1993. *Surpassing ourselves: An inquiry into the nature and implications of expertise.* La Salle, IL: Open Court.

———. 2003. Learning to work creatively with knowledge. In *Powerful learning environments: Unravelling basic components and dimensions,* ed. E. De Corte, L. Verschaffel, N. Entwistle, and J. van Merrienboer, 55–68. Oxford: Elsevier Science.

Berk, R. A. 1980. A consumers' guide to criterion-referenced test reliability. *Journal of Educational Measurement* 17 (4): 323–349.

Bhaba, H. 1987. Interrogating identity. In *Identity,* ed. L. Appignaesi, 5–11. London: Institute of Contemporary Art.

Bjork, R. A. 1999. Assessing our own competence: Heuristics and illusions. In *Attention and performance XVII: Cognitive regulation of performance,* ed. D. Gopher and A. Koriat, 435–459. Cambridge, MA: MIT Press.

Blanchette, I., and A. Richards. 2003. Anxiety and the interpretation of ambiguous information: Beyond the emotion-congruent effect. *Journal of Experimental Psychology: General* 132 (2): 294–309.

Bleakley, A. 2006. Broadening conceptions of learning in medical education: The message from teamworking. *Medical Education* 40:150–157.

Bleakley, A., and J. Bligh. 2007. Looking forward-looking back: Aspects of the contemporary debate about teaching and learning medicine. *Medical Teacher* 29:79–82.

Bleakley, A., J. Bligh, and J. Browne. 2010. *Medical education for the future: Identity, power and location.* Dordrecht: Springer.

Bleakley, A., J. Brice, and J. Bligh. 2008. Thinking the post-colonial in medical education. *Medical Education* 42:266–270.

Boehler, M. L., D. A. Rogers, C. J. Schwind, R. Mayforth, J. Quin, R. G. Williams, and G. Dunnington. 2006. An investigation of medical student response to feedback: A randomized controlled trial. *Medical Education* 40:746–749.

Boler, M. 1999. *Feeling power: Emotions and education.* New York: Routledge.

Bolhuis, S., and R.-J. Simons. 2003. Naar een breder begrip van leren [Toward a broader understanding of learning]. In *Human resource development: Organiseren van het leren* [Human resource development: Organizing learning], ed. J. W. M. Kessels and R. F. Poell, 37–52. Groningen: Samsom.

Bong, C. L., J. R. Lightdale, M. E. Fredette, and P. Weinstock. 2010. Effects of simulation versus traditional tutorial-based training on physiologic stress levels among clinicians: A pilot study. *Simulation in Healthcare* 5 (5): 272–278.

Bordage, G., and M. Lemieux. 1991. Semantic structures and diagnostic thinking of experts and novices. *Academic Medicine* 66 (9 suppl.): S70–S72.

Borrell-Carrio, F., and R. M. Epstein. 2004. Preventing errors in clinical practice: A call for self-awareness. *Annals of Family Medicine* 2 (4): 310–316.

Boud, D. 1999. Avoiding the traps: Seeking good practice in the use of self assessment and reflection in professional courses. *Social Work Education* 18:121–132.

Branch, W. T., R. Frankel, C. F. Gracey, P. M. Haidet, P. F. Weissmann, P. Cantey, G. A. Mitchell, and T. S. Inui. 2009. A good clinician and a caring person: Longitudinal faculty development and the enhancement of the human dimensions of care. *Academic Medicine* 84 (1): 117–125.

Branch, W. T., and T. K. Malik. 1993. Using "windows of opportunities" in brief interviews to understand patients' concerns. *Journal of the American Medical Association* 269 (13): 1667–1668.

Brand, J. E., and G. M. Stratton 1905. The effect of verbal suggestion upon the estimation of linear magnitudes. *Psychological Review* 12:41–49.

Bransford, J. 2000. *How people learn: Brain, mind, experience, and school.* Ed. National Research Council, Committee on Developments in the Science of Learning, and National Research Council, Committee on Learning Research and Educational Practice. Expanded ed. Washington, DC: National Academy Press.

Bransford, J. D., A. L. Brown, and R. R. Cocking. 2000. *How people learn.* Washington, DC: National Academy Press.

Bransford, J. D., and D. L. Schwartz. 1999. Rethinking transfer: A simple proposal with multiple implications. *Review of Research in Education* 24:61–100.

Brawer, J. 2009. Medical education: Striving for mediocrity. *Medical Education* 43:1026–1027.

Brooks, M. A. 2009. Medical education and the tyranny of competency. *Perspectives in Biology and Medicine* 52:90–102.

Brosnan, C., and B. Turner. 2009. *Handbook of the sociology of medical education.* London: Routledge.

Brown, J. S., A. Collins, and P. Duguid. 1989. Situated cognition and the culture of learning. *Educational Researcher* 18 (1): 32–42.

Brown, J. S., and P. Duguid. 1996. Organizational learning and communities-of-practice. In *Organizational learning,* ed. M. Cohen and L. Sproull, 48–82. London: Sage.

Bruer, J. T. 1997. Education and the brain: A bridge too far. *Educational Researcher* 26 (8): 1–13.

Buckman, R. 2005. Breaking bad news: The S-P-I-K-E-S strategy. *Psychosocial Oncology* (April): 138–142.

Burke, K. 1935. *Permanence and change.* New York: New Republic.

——. 1952. *A grammar of motives.* New York: Prentice Hall.

——. 1966. *Language as symbolic action: Essays on life, literature and method.* Berkeley: University of California Press.

——. 1968. *Counter-Statement.* Berkeley: University of California Press.

Butler, J. 2005. *Giving an account of oneself.* New York: Fordham University Press.

Butler, R. 1987. Task-involving and ego-involving properties of evaluation: Effects of different feedback conditions on motivational perceptions, interest, and performance. *Journal of Educational Psychology* 79:474–482.

Calhoun, C. 1995. *Critical social theory: Culture, history and the challenge of difference.* Oxford: Blackwell.

Canadian Institution of Healthcare Research (CIHR). 2006. Training tomorrow's health researchers today: CIHR's interdisciplinary training programs. http://www.cihr-irsc.gc.ca/e/30227.html (accessed January 28, 2010).

Canadian Medical Protective Association. 2008. Collaborative care: A medical liability perspective. http://www.cmpa-acpm.ca/cmpapd04/docs/submissions_papers/com_collaborative_care-e.cfm (accessed May 9, 2010).

Carraccio, C., S. D. Wolfsthal, R. Englander, K. Ferentz, and C. Martin. 2002. Shifting paradigms: From flexner to competencies. *Academic Medicine* 77:361–367.

Carrothers, R. M., S. W. Gregory, and T. J. Gallagher. 2000. Measuring emotional intelligence of medical school applicants. *Academic Medicine* 75:456–461.

Casson, R. W. 1983. Schema in cognitive anthropology. *Annual Review of Anthropology* 12:429–462.

Cathell, D. W. 1890. *Book on the physician himself.* Philadelphia: F. A. Davis.

Cervone, D. 2000. Thinking about self-efficacy. *Behavior Modification* 24:30–56.

Chalmers, A. F. 1999. *What is this thing called science?* Berkshire: Open University Press, McGraw Hill.

Charlin, B., H. P. Boshuizen, E. J. Custers, and P. J. Feltovich. 2007. Scripts and clinical reasoning. *Medical Education* 41 (12): 1178–1184.

Chi, M. T. H., P. J. Feltovich, and R. Glase. 1981. Categorization and representation physics problems by experts and novices. *Cognitive Science* 5:121–152.

Colby, A., and W. Sullivan. 2008. Formation of professionalism and purpose: Perspectives from the preparation for the professions program. *University of St. Thomas Law Journal* 5:404–428.

College of Physicians and Surgeons of Ontario. 2008. *Physician behaviour in the professional environment.* Policy statement 4-07. www.cpso.on.ca/policy.

Collins, J. P., I. R. Gough, I. D. Civil, and R. W. Stitz. 2007. New surgical education and training programme. *ANZ Journal of Surgery* 77:497–501.

Colliver, J. A., S. J. Verhulst, and H. S. Barrows. 2005. Self-assessment in medical practice: A further concern about the conventional research paradigm. *Teaching and Learning in Medicine* 17:200–201.

Connor, C. E., H. E. Egeth, and S. Yantis. 2004. Visual attention: Bottom-up versus top-down. *Current Biology* 14 (19): R850–R852.

Conway, A. R., M. J. Kane, M. F. Bunting, D. Z. Hambrick, O. Wilhelm, and R. W. Engle. 2005. Working memory span tasks: A methodological review and user's guide. *Psychonomic Bulletin and Review* 12 (5): 769–786.

Cook, S., and D. Yanow. 1993. Cultural and organizational learning. *Journal of Management Inquiry* 2:373–390.

Corbetta, M., and G. L. Shulman. 2002. Control of goal-directed and stimulus-driven attention in the brain. *Nature Review Neuroscience* 3 (3): 201–215.

Costello, C. Y. 2005. *Professional identity crisis: Race, class, gender, and success at professional schools.* Nashville: Vanderbilt University Press.

Cowan, N., E. M. Elliott, J. S. Saults, C. C. Morey, S. Mattox, A. Hismjatullina, and A. R. Conway. 2005. On the capacity of attention: Its estimation and its role in working memory and cognitive aptitudes. *Cognitive Psychology* 51 (1): 42–100.

Cronbach, L. J. 1951. Coefficient alpha and the internal structure of tests. *Psychometrika* 16:297–334.

Cronbach, L. J., and P. E. Meehl. 1955. Construct validity in psychological tests. *Psychological Bulletin* 52 (4): 281–303.

Cronbach, L. J., and R. J. Shavelson. 2004. My current thoughts on coefficient alpha and successor procedures. *Educational and Psychological Measurement* 64 (3): 391–418.

Csikszentmihalyi, M., and I. S. Csikszentmihalyi. 2000. *Beyond boredom and anxiety: Experiencing flow in work and play.* San Francisco: Jossey-Bass.

Custers, E. J. F. M., G. Regehr, and G. R. Norman. 1996. Mental representations of medical diagnostic knowledge: A review. *Academic Medicine* 71 (10): S55–S61.

Dainty, A. R. J., M. I. Cheng, and D. R. Moore. 2005. Competency-based model for predicting construction project managers' performance. *Journal of Management in Engineering* 21:2–5.

Dalgleish, T. 2004. The emotional brain. *Nature Reviews Neuroscience* 5:582–589.

Damasio, A. R. 1994. *Descartes' error: Emotion, reason, and the human brain.* New York: G. P. Putnam.

———. 1997. Towards a neuropathology of emotion and mood. *Nature* 386:769–770.

———. 1999. *The feeling of what happens: Body and emotion in the making of consciousness.* New York: Harcourt Brace.

Damasio, A. R., B. J. Everitt, and D. Bishop. 1996. The somatic marker hypothesis and the possible functions of the prefrontal cortex. *Philosophical Transactions: Biological Sciences* 351 (1346): 1413–1420.

Darwin, C. 1872. *The expression of the emotions in man and animals.* London: Murray.

Davis, D. A., P. E. Mazmanian, M. Fordis, R. Van Harrison, K. E. Thorpe, and L. Perrier. 2006. Accuracy of physician self-assessment compared with observed measures of competence: A systematic review. *Journal of the American Medical Association* 296:1094–1102.

DelVecchio Good, M.-J. 1995. *American medicine: The quest for competence.* Berkeley: University of California Press.

Descartes, R. 1649. *Passions of the soul.* Trans. and annotated Stephen Voss. Indianapolis: Hackett, 1989.

De Souza, C., and M. Solomon. 2009. A novel approach to teaching communication: Using the Cognitive Behavioral Model (CBM). *Poster proceedings for the American Association of Academic Psychiatry Washington D.C.*

Dobson, K., and R.-L. Franche. 1989. A conceptual and empirical review of the depressive realism hypothesis. *Canadian Journal of Behavioural Science* 21:419–433.

Dolan, R. J. 2002. Emotion, cognition, and behavior. *Science* 298 (5596): 1191–1194.

Dornhorst, A. C. 1981. Information overload: Why medical education needs a shakeup. *Lancet* 2:513–514.

Dowdle, M. W. 2006. *Public accountability: Designs, dilemmas and experiences.* Cambridge: Cambridge University Press.

Dreyfus, H. L., T. Athanasiou, and S. E. Dreyfus. 1986. *Mind over machine: The power of human intuition and expertise in the era of the computer.* New York: Free Press.

Driessen, E., C. P. M. van der Vleuten, L. W. T. Schuwirth, J. van Tartwijk, and J. Vermunt. 2005. The use of qualitative research criteria for portfolio assessment as an alternative to reliability evaluation: A case study. *Medical Education* 39 (2): 214–220.

Driskell, J. E., J. H. Johnston, and E. Salas. 2001. Does stress training generalize to novel settings? *Human Factors* 43:99–110.

Dryburgh, H. 1999. Work hard, play hard: Women and professionalization in engineering; Adapting to the culture. *Gender & Society* 13 (5): 664–682.

Dryer, B. V. 1961. Lifetime learning for physicians: Principles, practices, proposals. *Journal of Medical Education* 37 (part 2): 1–134.

Dunning, D., C. Heath, and J. M. Suls. 2004. Flawed self-assessment: Implications for health, education, and the workplace. *Psychological Science in the Public Interest* 5:69–106.

Dweck, C. S. 1999. Caution: Praise can be dangerous. *American Educator* (Spring): 1–5.

Dyche, L., and R. M. Epstein. 2011. Curiosity and medical education. *Medical Education* 45 (7): 663–668.

Economist. 2007. International: Great plot, shame about the characters; Psychiatry and films. March 24–30, 77.

Elam, C., T. D. Stratton, and M. A. Andrykowski. 2001. Measuring the emotional intelligence of medical school matriculants. *Academic Medicine* 76:507–508.

Elias, N. 1978. *The Civilizing Process: The History of Manners,* trans. E. Jephcott, Oxford: Blackwell.

Elstein, A. S., A. Schwartz, J. Higgs, and M. Jones. 2000. Clinical reasoning in medicine. In *Clinical reasoning in the health professions,* ed. J. Higgs, M. Jones, S. Loftus, and N. Christensen, 223–234. Oxford: Butterworth Heinemann.

Elstein, A. S., L. S. Shulman, and S. A. Sprafka. 1978. *Medical problem solving: An analysis of clinical reasoning.* Cambridge, MA: Harvard University Press.

Endsley, M. R. 1995. Toward a theory of situation awareness in dynamic-systems. *Human Factors* 37 (1): 32–64.

Engeström, Y. 1987. *Learning by expanding: An activity-theoretical approach to developmental research.* Helsinki: Orienta-Konsultit.

———. 2000. Activity theory as a framework for analyzing and redesigning work. *Ergonomics* 43:960–974.

———. 2001. Expansive learning at work: Toward an activity theoretical reconceptualization. *Journal of Education and Work* 14 (1): 133–156.

Epictetus. Circa 135. *Discourses.* http://en.wikiquote.org/wiki/Epictetus.

Epstein, R. 1999. Mindful practice. *Journal of the American Medical Association* 282:833–839.

———. 2003a. Mindful practice in action (I): Technical competence, evidence-based medicine, and relationship-centered care. *Families, Systems, & Health* 21 (1): 1–9.

———. 2003b. Mindful practice in action (II): Cultivating habits of mind. *Families, Systems, & Health* 21 (1): 11–17.

Epstein, R. M., D. J. Siegel, and J. Silberman. 2008. Self-monitoring in clinical practice: A challenge for medical educators. *Journal of Continuing Education in the Health Professions* 28:5–13.

Epstein, R. M., and R. L. Street. 2011. Shared minds: Collaborative decision-making in serious illness. *Annals of Family Medicine* 9 (5): 454–461.

Eraut, M. 1994. *Developing professional knowledge and competence.* London: Falmer Press.

———. 2000. Non-formal learning and tacit knowledge in professional work. *British Journal of Educational Psychology* 70:113–136.

Ericsson, K. A., R. T. Krampe, and C. Teschromer. 1993. The role of deliberate practice in the acquisition of expert performance. *Psychological Review* 100 (3): 363–406.

Eva, K. W. 2001. Assessing tutorial-based assessment. *Advances in Health Sciences Education* 6:243–257.

———. 2002. The aging physician: Changes in cognitive processing and their impact on medical practice. *Academic Medicine* 77 (10): S1–S6.

———. 2003. On the generality of specificity. *Medical Education* 37 (7): 587–588.

———. 2005. What every teacher needs to know about clinical reasoning. *Medical Education* 39:98–106.

———. 2007. Putting the cart before the horse: Testing to improve learning. *British Medical Journal* 334:535.

———. 2009. Diagnostic error in medical education: Where wrongs can make rights. *Advances in Health Sciences Education* 14:71–81.

Eva, K. W., H. Armson, E. Holmboe, J. Lockyer, E. Loney, K. V. Mann, and J. M. Sargeant. 2011. Factors influencing responsiveness to feedback: On the interplay between fear, confidence, and reasoning processes. *Advances in Health Sciences Education* (April 6). doi:10.1007/s10459-011-9290-7, http://www.springerlink.com/content/k890327358w37521/.

Eva, K. W., J. P. W. Cunnington, H. I. Reiter, D. R. Keane, and G. R. Norman. 2004. How can I know what I don't know? Poor self-assessment in a well-defined domain. *Advances in Health Sciences Education* 9:211–224.

Eva, K. W., R. M. Hatala, V. R. LeBlanc, and L. R. Brooks. 2007. Teaching from the clinical reasoning literature: Combined reasoning strategies help novice diagnosticians overcome misleading information. *Medical Education* 41:1152–1158.

Eva, K. W., J. Munoz, M. D. Hanson, A. Walsh, and J. Wakefield. 2010. Which factors, personal or external, most influence students' generation of learning goals? *Academic Medicine* 85:S102–S105.

Eva, K. W., and G. R. Norman. 2005. Heuristics and biases: A biased perspective on clinical reasoning. *Medical Education* 39 (9): 870–872.

Eva, K. W., and G. Regehr. 2005. Self-assessment in the health professions: A reformulation and research agenda. *Academic Medicine* 80 (10 suppl): S46–S54.

———. 2007. Knowing when to look it up: A new conception of self-assessment ability. *Academic Medicine* 82:S81–S84.

———. 2008. "I'll never play professional football" and other fallacies of self-assessment. *Journal for Continuing Education in the Health Professions* 28:14–19.

———. 2011. Exploring the divergence between self-assessment and self-monitoring. *Advances in Health Sciences Education* 16:311–329.

Farb, N. A., Z. V. Segal, H. Mayberg, J. Bean, D. McKeon, Z. Fatima, and A. K. Anderson. 2007. Attending to the present: Mindfulness meditation reveals distinct neural modes of self-reference. *Social Cognitive and Affective Neuroscience* 2 (4): 313–322.

Farnsworth, W. E. 1991. Training physicians to be doctors—teachers and healers, problem-solvers and decision-makers. *Journal of the American Osteopathic Association* 91:1005–1001.

Feinstein, A. R. 1994. "Clinical judgment" revisited: The distraction of quantitative models. *Annals of Internal Medicine* 120 (9): 799–805.

Feldman, M. D. 2001. Becoming an emotionally intelligent physician. *Western Journal of Medicine* 175 (2): 98.

Fioratou, E., R. Flin, R. Glavin, and R. Patey. 2010. Beyond monitoring: Distributed situation awareness in anaesthesia. *British Journal of Anaesthesia* 105 (1): 83–90.

Fitzgerald, J. T., C. B. White, and L. D. Gruppen. 2003. A longitudinal study of self-assessment accuracy. *Medical Education* 37:645–649.

Fitzsimmons, G. M., and E. J. Finkel. 2011. Outsourcing self-regulation. *Psychological Science* 22:369–375.

Flavell, J. H. 1976. Metacognitive aspects of problem solving. In *The nature of intelligence,* ed. L. B. Resnick, 231–236. Hillsdale, NJ: Erlbaum.

———. 1979. Metacognition and cognitive monitoring: A new area of cognitive-developmental inquiry. *American Psychologist* 34:906–911.

Flexner, A. 1910. *Medical education in the United States and Canada: A report to the Carnegie Foundation for the Advancement of Teaching.* Bulletin no. 4. Boston: Updyke.

Folk, C. L., and R. Remington. 2006. Top-down modulation of preattentive processing: Testing the recovery account of contingent capture. *Visual Cognition* 14 (4–8): 445–465.

Foucault, M. 1977. *Discipline and punish: The birth of the prison.* New York: Vintage Books.

———. 1980. *An introduction.* Vol. 1 of *The history of sexuality.* Trans. R. Hurley. New York: Random House, 1980.

———. 1990. *The use of pleasure.* Vol. 2 of *The history of sexuality.* Trans. R. Hurley. New York: Vintage Books.

Foy, R., M. Eccles, G. Jamtvedt, J. Young, J. M. Grimshaw, and R. Baker. 2005. What do we know about how to do audit and feedback? Pitfalls in applying evidence from a systematic review. *BMC Health Services Research* 5:50.

Frank, J. R., ed. 2005. *The CanMEDS 2005 physician competency framework: Better standards, better physicians, better care.* Ottawa: The Royal College of Physicians and Surgeons of Canada.

Frank, J. R., L. S. Snell, O. ten Cate, E. S. Holmboe, C. Carraccio, S. R. Swing, P. Harris, et al. 2010. Competency-based medical education: Theory to practice. *Medical Teacher* 32:638–645.

Friedrich, J. 1996. On seeing oneself as less self-serving than others: The ultimate self-serving bias? *Teaching of Psychology* 23:107–109.

Fullerton, J. T., A. Bherissi, P. G. Johnson, and J. B. Thompson. 2001. Competence and competency: Core concepts for international midwifery practice. *International Journal of Childbirth* 1:4–12.

Gaab, J., N. Blättler, T. Menzi, B. Pabst, S. Stoyer, and U. Ehlert. 2003. Randomized controlled evaluation of the effects of cognitive-behavioral stress management on cortisol responses to acute stress in healthy subjects. *Psychoneuroendocrinology* 28:767–779.

Gaab, J., L. Sonderegger, S. Scherrer, and U. Ehlert. 2006. Psychoneuroendocrine effects of cognitive-behavioral stress management in a naturalistic setting: A randomized controlled trial. *Psychoneuroendocrinology* 31:428–438.

Gailliot, M. T., E. Ashby Plant, D. A. Butz, and R. F. Baumeister. 2007. Increasing self-regulatory strength can reduce the depleting effect of suppressing stereotypes. *Personality and Social Psychology Bulletin* 33 (2): 281–294.

Galbraith, R. M., R. E. Hawkins, and E. S. Holmboe. 2008. Making self-assessment more effective. *Journal of Continuing Education in the Health Professions* 28:20–24.

Gallese, V., C. Keysers, and G. Rizzolatti. 2004. A unifying view of the basis of social cognition. *Trends in Cognitive Sciences* 8 (9): 396–403.

Garavan, T. N., and D. McGuire. 2001. Competencies and workplace learning: Some reflections on the rhetoric and the reality. *Journal of Workplace Learning* 13:144–164.

Gardner, H. 1985. *The mind's new science.* New York: Basic Books.

Garofalo, J. 1986. Metacognitive knowledge and metacognitive process: Important influences on mathematical performance. *Research and Training in Developmental Education* 2:34–39.

Gawande, A. A., M. J. Zinner, D. M. Studdert, and T. A. Brennan. 2003. Analysis of errors reported by surgeons at three teaching hospitals. *Surgery* 133:614–621.

Gendron, M., and L. F. Barrett. 2009. Reconstructing the past: A century of ideas about emotion in psychology. *Emotion Review* 1 (4): 316–339.

General Medical Council. 1993. *Tomorrow's doctors: Recommendations on undergraduate medical education.* London: General Medical Council.

———. 2010. The role of the GMC. http://www.gmc-uk.org/about/role.asp (accessed March 10, 2010).

Gergen, K. J., and K. E. Davis. 1985. *The social construction of the person.* Springer Series in Social Psychology. New York: Springer-Verlag.

Germer, C. K., R. D. Siegel, and P. R. Fulton. 2005. *Mindfulness and psychotherapy.* New York: Guilford Press.

Gick, M. L., and K. J. Holyoak. 1980. Analogical problem solving. *Cognitive Psychology* 12:306–355.

Gieryn, T. F., G. M. Bevins, and S. C. Zehr. 1985. Professionalization of American scientists: Public science in the creation/evolution trials. *American Sociological Review* 50:392–409.

Gigerenzer, G. 2007. *Gut feelings: The intelligence of the unconscious.* New York: Viking.

Gilbert, D. T., and T. D. Wilson. 2000. Miswanting. In *Thinking and feeling: The role of affect in social cognition,* ed. J. Forgas, 178–197. Cambridge: Cambridge University Press.

Gilovich, T. 1991. *How we know what isn't so: The fallibility of human reason in everyday life.* New York: The Free Press.

Ginsburg, S., J. McIlroy, O. Oulanova, K. Eva, and G. Regehr. 2010. Towards authentic clinical evaluation: Pitfalls in the pursuit of competency. *Medical Education* 85:780–786.

Ginsburg, S., G. Regehr, and L. Lingard. 2003. The disavowed curriculum: Understanding students' reasoning in professionally challenging situations. *Journal of General Internal Medicine* 18:1015–1022.

——. 2004. Basing the assessment of professionalism on observable behaviors: A cautionary tale. *Academic Medicine* 79:S1–S4.

Glass, D. C., and J. D. McKnight. 1996. Perceived control, depressive symptomatology, and professional burnout: A review of evidence. *Psychology and Health* 11:1, 23–48.

Godkins, T. R., D. Duffy, J. Greenwood, and W. D. Stanhope. 1974. Utilization of simulated patients to teach the "routine" pelvic examination. *Journal of Medical Education* 49:1174–1178.

Goffman, E. 1959. *The presentation of self in everyday life.* London: Doubleday.

Goldman, G. M. 1990. The tacit dimension of clinical judgment. *Yale Journal of Biology and Medicine* 63 (1): 47–61.

Goleman, D. 1995. *Emotional intelligence: Why it can matter more than IQ.* New York: Bantam Books.

Goleman, D., and R. Boyatz. 2008. Social intelligence and the biology of leadership. *Growth: Journal of the Management Training Institute* 36 (2): 52–55.

Gordon, C. 1980. *Power/knowledge: Selected interviews and other writings, 1972–1977, by Michel Foucault.* New York: Pantheon Books.

Gordon, D. 1988. Tenacious assumptions in Western medicine. In *Biomedicine examined,* ed. M. Lock and D. Gordon, 19–56. Dordrecht: Kluwer Academic.

Gordon, M. J. 1991. A review of the validity and accuracy of self-assessments in health professions training. *Academic Medicine* 66:762–769.

——. 1992. Self-assessment programs and their implications for health professions training. *Academic Medicine* 67:672–679.

Gott, S., P. Hall, A. Pokorny, E. Dibble, and R. Glaser. 1992. A naturalistic study of transfer: Adaptive expertise in technical domains. In *Transfer on trial: Intelligence, cognition, and instruction,* ed. D. Detterman and R. Sternberg, 258–288. Norwood, NJ: Ablex.

Govaerts, M. J. B., L. W. T. Schuwirth, C. P. M. van der Vleuten, and A. M. M. Mui-jtjens. 2011. Workplace-based assessment: Effects of rater expertise. *Advances in Health Sciences Education* 16 (2): 151–165.

Govaerts, M. J. B., C. P. M. van der Vleuten, L. W. T. Schuwirth, and A. M. M. Mui-jtjens 2007. Broadening perspectives on clinical performance assessment: Rethinking the nature of in-training assessment. *Advances in Health Sciences Education* 12 (2): 239–260.

Grant, G. 1979. *On competence: A critical analysis of competence-based reforms in higher education.* San Francisco: Jossey-Bass.

Grant, G., and C. E. Murray. 1999. *Teaching in America: The slow revolution.* Cambridge, MA: Harvard University Press.

Grantcharov, T. P., and R. K. Reznick. 2009. Training tomorrow's surgeons: What are we looking for and how can we achieve it? *ANZ Journal of Surgery* 79:104–107.

Greene, M. 1973. *Teacher as stranger.* Belmont, CA: Wadsworth.

Greeno, J. G., D. R. Smith, and J. L. Moore. 1993. Transfer of situated learning. In *Transfer on trial: Intelligence, cognition, and instruction,* ed. D. K. Detterman and R. J. Sternberg, 99–167. Westport, CT: Ablex.

Gros, C. 2010. Cognition and emotion: Perspectives on a closing gap. *Cognitive Computation* 2 (2): 78–85.

Gross, J. J. 2002. Emotion regulation: Affective, cognitive and social consequences. *Psychophysiology* 39:281–291.

Haber, R., and L. Lingard. 2001. Learning oral presentation skills: A rhetorical analysis with pedagogical and professional implications. *Journal of General Internal Medicine* 16:308–314.

Hafferty, F. W. 1991. *Into the valley: Death and the socialization of medical students.* New Haven, CT: Yale University Press.

———. 1998. Beyond curriculum reform: Confronting medicine's hidden curriculum. *Academic Medicine* 73:403–407.

Haidet, P., M. L. Fecile, H. F. West, and C. R. Teal. 2009. Reconsidering the team concept: Educational implications for patient-centered cancer care. *Patient Education and Counseling* 77 (3): 450–455.

Hall, S. 1997. *Representation: Cultural representations and signifying practices.* London: Sage.

Hambleton, R. K., and M. R. Novik. 1973. Toward an integration of theory and method for criterion-referenced tests. *Journal of Educational Measurement* 10 (3): 159–170.

Hambleton, R. K., H. Swaminathan, J. Algina, and D. B. Coulson. 1978. Criterion-referenced testing and measurement: A review of technical issues and developments. *Review of Educational Research* 48 (1): 1–47.

Hammerfald, K., C. Eberle, and M. Grau. 2006. Persistent effects of cognitive-behavioral stress management on cortisol responses to acute stress in health subjects: A randomized controlled trial. *Psychoneuroendocrinology* 31:333–339.

Handfield-Jones, R. S., K. V. Mann, M. E. Challis, S. O. Hobma, D. J. Klass, I. C. McManus, N. S. Paget, I. J. Parboosingh, W. B. Wade, and T. J. Wilkinson. 2002. Linking assessment to learning: A new route to quality assurance in medical practice. *Medical Education* 36:949–958.

Hanna, M., and J. Fins. 2006. Power and communication: Why simulation training ought to be complemented by experiential and humanist learning. *Academic Medicine* 81 (3): 265–270.

Hanson, F. A. 1993. *Testing testing: The social consequences of the examined life.* Berkeley: University of California Press.

Harvey, A., Bandiera, B., Nathens, A. B., LeBlanc, V. R. Forthcoming. The impact of stress on resident performance in simulated trauma scenarios. *Journal of Trauma, Injury, Infection and Critical Care.*

Harvey, A., A. B. Nathens, G. L. Bandiera, and V. R. LeBlanc. 2010. Threat and challenge: cognitive appraisal and stress responses in simulated trauma resuscitations. *Medical Education* 44 (6): 587–594.

Hatano, G., and K. Inagaki. 1986. Two courses of expertise. In *Child development and education in Japan,* ed. H. Stevenson, H. Azuma, and K. Hakuta, 262–272. New York: W. H. Freeman.

Hattie, J., and H. Timperley. 2007. The power of feedback. *Review of Educational Research* 77:81–112.

Haynes, A. B., T. G. Weiser, W. R. Berry, S. R. Lipsitz, A. H. S. Breizat, E. P. Dellinger, T. Herbosa, et al. 2009. A surgical safety checklist to reduce morbidity and mortality in a global population. *New England Journal of Medicine* 360:491.

Hays, R., and S. Gay. 2011. Reflection or "pre-reflection": What are we actually measuring in reflective practice? *Medical Education* 45:116–118.

Health Canada. 2010. Creating healthy, supportive, learning workplaces. http://www.hc-sc.gc.ca/hcs-sss/hhr-rhs/strateg/p3/index-eng.php (accessed July 6, 2011).

Hein, K. 2010. The competency of competencies. *Prehospital & Disaster Medicine* 25:396–397.

Higgins, E. T. 1997. Beyond pleasure and pain. *American Psychologist* 52:1280–1300.

———. 1998. Promotion and prevention: Regulatory focus as a motivational principle. *Advances in Experimental Social Psychology* 30:1–46.

Ho, M. J., K. Yu, D. Hirsh, T. Huang, and P. C. Yang. 2011. Does one size fit all? Building a framework for medical professionalism. *Academic Medicine* 86:1407–1414.

Hochschild, A. R. 2003. *The managed heart: Commercialization of human feeling.* Berkeley: University of California Press.

Hodges, B. D. 2003. OSCE! Variations on a theme by Harden. *Medical Education* 37:1134–1140.

———. 2004. Medical student bodies and the pedagogy of self-reflection, self-assessment and self-regulation. *Journal of Curriculum Theorizing* 20:41–51.

———. 2005. The many and conflicting histories of medical education in Canada and the United States: An introduction to the paradigm wars. *Medical Education* 39:613–621.

———. 2006. Medical education and the maintenance of incompetence. *Medical Teacher* 28:690–696.

———. 2007. A socio-historical study of the birth and adoption of the Objective Structured Clinical Examination (OSCE). PhD diss., Ontario Institute for Studies in Education.

———. 2009. *The objective structured clinical examination: A socio-history.* Cologne: LAP Lambert Academic.

———. 2010. Clinical commentary. In *My imaginary illness: A journey into uncertainty and prejudice in medical diagnosis,* ed. C. G. K. Atkins, 153–192. Ithaca, NY: Cornell University Press.

Hodges, B. D., J. M. Maniate, M. A. Matimianakis, M. Alsuwaidan, and C. Segouin. 2009. Cracks and crevices: Globalization discourse and medical education. *Medical Teacher* 31:910–917.

Hodges, B. D., G. Regehr, and D. Martin. 2001. Difficulties in recognizing one's own incompetence: Novice physicians who are unskilled and unaware of it. *Academic Medicine* 76:S87–S89.

Hodges, B. D., G. Regehr, N. McNaughton, R. Tiberius, and M. Hanson. 1999. OSCE checklists do not capture increasing levels of expertise. *Academic Medicine* 74:64–69.

Hong, Y. Y., M. W. Morris, C. Y. Chiu, and V. Benet-Martinez. 2000. Multicultural minds: A dynamic constructivist approach to culture and cognition. *American Psychologist* 55 (7): 709–720.

Horowitz, S. D., S. H. Miller, and P. V. Miles. 2004. Board certification and physician quality. *Medical Education* 38:1364–1365.

Houston, R. W. 1973. Designing competency-based instructional systems. *Journal of Teacher Education* 24:200–204.

Hsu, K. E., F. Y. Man, R. A. Gizicki, L. S. Feldman, and G. M. Fried. 2008. Experienced surgeons can do more than one thing at a time: Effect of distraction on performance of a simple laparoscopic and cognitive task by experienced and novice surgeons. *Surgical Endoscopy* 22 (1): 196–201.

Huddle T. S., and G. R. Heudebert. 2007. Taking apart the art: The risk of anatomizing clinical competence. *Academic Medicine* 82:536–541.

Hume, D. 1739–1740. *A treatise on human nature.* New York: E. P. Dutton, 1911.

Hutchins, E. 1993. Learning to navigate. In *Understanding practice: Perspectives on activity and context,* ed. by S. Chaiklin & J. Lave, 35–63. Cambridge: Cambridge University Press.

———. 1995. *Cognition in the wild.* Cambridge, MA: MIT Press.

———. 1995. How a cockpit remembers its speed. *Cognitive Science* 19 (3): 265–288.

Hutchins, E., and T. Klausen. 1998. Distributed cognition in an airline cockpit. In *Cognition and communication at work,* ed. Y. Engeström and D. Middleton, 15–34. New York: Cambridge University Press.

Iedema, R., and H. Scheeres. 2003. From doing work to talking work: Renegotiating knowing, doing and identity. *Applied Linguistics* 24:316–337.

Institute for International Medical Education (Core Committee). 2002. Global minimum essential requirements in medical education. *Medical Teacher* 24:130–135.

Izard, C. E. 2009. Emotion theory and research: Highlights, unanswered questions and emerging issues. *Annual Review of Psychology* 60:1–15.

Jackson, M. 1988. Man in the mirror. http://en.wikipedia.org/wiki/Man_in_the_Mirror (accessed November 28, 2011).

Jefferies, A., B. Simmons, E. Ng, and M. Skidmore. 2011. Assessment of multiple physician competencies in postgraduate training: Utility of the structured oral examination. *Advances in Health Sciences Education* 16:569–577.

Jin, J., M. Martimianakis, S. Kitto, and C. A. Moulton. Forthcoming. Pressures to "measure up" in surgery: Managing your image and managing your patient. *Annals of Surgery.*

Johnston, J. H., and J. A. Cannon-Bowers. 1996. Training for stress exposure. In *Stress and human performance,* ed. J. E. Driskell and E. Salas, 223–279. Mahwah, NJ: Lawrence Erlbaum Associates.

Joint Commission on Accreditation of Healthcare Organizations (JCAHO). 2005. *Sentinel event statistics: December 17, 2003.* Oakbrook Terrace, IL: JCAHO.

Jones, D. G., and M. R. Endsley. 1996. Sources of situation awareness errors in aviation. *Aviation Space and Environmental Medicine* 67 (6): 507–512.

Kabat-Zinn, J. 2005. Bringing mindfulness to medicine: An interview with Jon Kabat-Zinn, PhD. Interview by Karolyn Gazella. *Advances in Mind-Body Medicine* 21 (2): 22–27.

Kahneman, D. 1973. *Attention and effort.* Prentice-Hall Series in Experimental Psychology. Englewood Cliffs, NJ: Prentice-Hall.

Kahneman, D., P. Slovic, and A. Tversky. 1982. *Judgment under uncertainty: Heuristics and biases.* Cambridge: Cambridge University Press.

Kane, M. T. 2006. Validation. In *Educational measurement,* ed. R. L. Brennan, 17–64. Westport, CT: ACE/Praeger.

Karle, H. 2006. Global standards and accreditation in medical education: A view from the WFME. *Academic Medicine* 81:S43–S48.

Kasper, D. 2005. *Harrison's principles of internal medicine.* New York: McGraw-Hill.

Kemper, T. D. 1993. Sociological models in the explanation of emotions. In *Handbook of emotions,* ed. M. Lewis and J. M. Haviland, 41–51. New York: Guilford Press.

Kennedy, T. J., G. Regehr, R. Baker, and L. A. Lingard. 2009. "It's a cultural expectation…": The pressure on medical trainees to work independently in clinical practice. *Medical Education* 43:645–653.

Kensinger, E. A. 2009. Remembering the details: Effects of emotions. *Emotion Review* 1 (2): 99–113.

Kierkegaard, S. A. 1841. Irony as a mastered moment: The truth of irony. Part 2 of The concept of irony. Thesis, University of Copenhagen.

Kim, M. S., and K. R. Cave. 1999. Top-down and bottom-up attentional control: On the nature of interference from a salient distractor. *Perception & Psychophysics* 61 (6): 1009–1023.

Kincheloe, J. L., and P. L. McLaren. 2000. Rethinking critical theory and qualitative research. In *Handbook of qualitative research,* ed. N. K. Denzin and Y. S. Lincoln, 138–157. Thousand Oaks, CA: Sage.

King, M. L. 1967. Where do we go from here? Speech delivered at the Southern Christian Leadership Conference, Atlanta.

Klass, D. 2007. A performance-based conception of competence is changing the regulation of physicians' professional behavior. *Academic Medicine* 82 (6): 529–535.

Klein, G. 1999. *Sources of power: How people make decisions.* Cambridge, MA: MIT Press.

Kluger, A. N., and A. DeNisi. 1996. The effects of feedback interventions on performance: A historical review, a meta-analysis, and a preliminary feedback intervention theory. *Psychological Bulletin* 119:254–284.

Kluger, A. N., and D. van Dijk. 2010. Feedback, the various tasks of the doctor, and the feedforward alternative. *Medical Education* 44:1166–1174.

Koriat, A., R. A. Bjork, L. Sheffer, and S. K. Bar. 2004. Predicting one's own forgetting: The role of experience-based and theory-based processes. *Journal of Experimental Psychology: General* 113:643–656.

Krasner, M. S., R. M. Epstein, H. Beckman, A. L. Suchman, B. Chapman, C. J. Mooney, and T. E. Quill. 2009. Association of an educational program in mindful communication with burnout, empathy, and attitudes among primary care physicians. *Journal of the American Medical Association* 302 (12): 1284–1293.

Kreps, G. L. 2009. Applying Weick's model of organizing to health care and health promotion: Highlighting the central role of health communication. *Patient Education and Counseling* 74 (3): 347–355.

Krieger, J. L. 2005. Shared mindfulness in cockpit crisis situations: An exploratory analysis. *Journal of Business Communication* 42 (2): 135–167.

Kromann, C. B., C. Bohnstedt, M. L. Jensen, and C. Ringsted. 2010. The testing effect on skills learning might last 6 months. *Advances in Health Sciences Education* 15:395–401.

Kromann, C. B., M. L. Jensen, and C. Ringsted. 2009. The effect of testing on skills learning. *Medical Education* 43:21–27.

Kruger, J., and D. Dunning. 1999. Unskilled and unaware of it: How difficulties in recognizing one's own incompetence lead to inflated self-assessments. *Journal of Personality and Social Psychology* 77:1121–1134.

Kuper, A., M. Albert, and B. D. Hodges. 2010. The origins of the field of medical education research. *Academic Medicine* 85:1347–1353.

Kuper, A., and B. D. Hodges. 2010. Medical education in societies. In *Medical education: Theory and practice,* ed. T. Dornan, K. V. Mann, A. J. J. A. Scherpbier, and J. A. Spencer, 39–49. London: Elsevier.

Kuper, A., S. Reeves, M. Albert, and B. D. Hodges. 2007. Assessment: Do we need to broaden our methodological horizons? *Medical Education* 41:1121–1123.

Kwolek-Folland, A. 1994. *Engendering business: Men and women in the corporate office, 1870–1930.* Berkeley: University of California Press.

Lamy, D., Y. Tsal, and H. Egeth. 2003. Does a salient distractor capture attention early in processing? *Psychonomic Bulletin and Review* 10 (3): 621–629.

Langer, E. J. 1997. *The power of mindful learning.* Reading, MA: Addison-Wesley.

Larsen, D. P., A. C. Butler, and H. L. Roediger. 2008. Test-enhanced learning in medical education. *Medical Education* 42:959–966.

Lave, J. 1988. *Cognition in practice.* Cambridge: Cambridge University Press.

———. 1991. Situating learning in communities of practice. In *Perspectives on socially shared cognition,* ed. L. Resnick, J. M. Levine, and S. D. Teasley, 63–82. Washington, DC: American Psychological Association.

Lave, J., and E. Wenger. 1991. *Situated learning: Legitimate peripheral participation.* New York: Cambridge University Press.

Lazar, S. W., C. E. Kerr, R. H. Wasserman, J. R. Gray, D. N. Greve, M. T. Treadway, M. McGarvey, et al. 2005. Meditation experience is associated with increased cortical thickness. *Neuroreport* 16 (17): 1893–1897.

Lazarus, R. S. 1991. *Emotion and adaptation.* New York: Oxford University Press.

LeBlanc, V. R., and G. Bandiera. 2007. The effects of examination stress on the performance of emergency medicine residents. *Medical Education* 41:556–564.

LeBlanc, V. R., R. D. MacDonald, B. McArthur, K. King, and T. Lepine. 2005. Paramedic performance in calculating drug dosages following stressful scenarios in a human patient simulator. *Prehospital Emergency Care* 9 (4): 439–444.

LeBlanc, V. R., G. R. Norman, and L. R. Brooks. 2001. Effect of a diagnostic suggestion on diagnostic accuracy and identification of clinical features. *Academic Medicine* 76 (10): S18–S20.

LeBlanc, V. R., W. Tavares, K. King, A. K. Scott, R. Macdonald, and C. Regehr. 2010. The impact of stress on paramedic performance during simulated critical events. *Simulation in Healthcare* 5 (6): 440.

LeBlanc, V. R., S. I. Woodrow, R. Sidhu, and A. Dubrowski. 2008. Examination stress leads to improvements on fundamental technical skills for surgery. *American Journal of Surgery* 196 (1): 114–119.

LeDoux, J. 1996. *The emotional brain: The mysterious underpinnings of emotional life.* New York: Simon & Schuster.

Lesser, M. 2009. *Less: Accomplishing more by doing less.* Novato, CA: New World Library.

Leung, A., S. Luu, G. Regehr, and C. A. Moulton. 2011. First do no harm: Balancing competing priorities in surgical practice. Unpublished manuscript.

Leung, W.-C. 2002. Competency based medical training: Review. *British Medical Journal* 325:693–695.

Lewis, N. J., C. E. Rees, J. N. Hudson, and A. Bleakley. 2005. Emotional intelligence in medical education: Measuring the unmeasurable? *Advances in Health Sciences Education* 10:339–355.

Liaison Committee on Medical Education. 2011. Accreditation standards for Canadian and American medical education programs. http://www. lcme.org/connections.htm (accessed December 6, 2011).

Lingard, L. 2009. What we see and don't see when we look at "competence": Notes on a god term. *Advances in Health Sciences Education Theory and Practice* 14 (5): 625–628.

Lingard, L., and R. J. Haber. 1999. What do we mean by "relevance"? A clinical and rhetorical definition with implications for teaching and learning the case presentation format. *Academic Medicine* 74:S124–S127.

Lingard, L., S. Whyte, G. Regehr, and F. Gardezi. 2009. Counting silence: Complexities in the evaluation of team communication. In *Safer surgery: Analysing behaviour in the operating theatre,* ed. R. Flin and L. Mitchell, 283–301. Burlington, VT: Ashgate.

Lloyd, F. J., and V. F. Reyna. 2009. Clinical gist and medical education: Connecting the dots. *Journal of the American Medical Association* 302 (12): 1332–1333.

Long, D. M. 2000. Competency-based residency training: The next advance in graduate medical education. *Academic Medicine* 75:1178–1183.

Lurie S. J., C. J. Mooney, and J. M. Lyness. 2009. Measurement of the general competencies of the Accreditation Council for Graduate Medical Education: A systematic review. *Academic Medicine* 84:301–309.

Lutz, C. 2007. Emotion, thought and estrangement: Emotion as a cultural category. In *The emotions: A cultural reader,* ed. H. Wulff, 21–35. Oxford: Berg.

Lutz, C., and L. Abu-Lughod. 1990. Emotion, discourse and the politics of everyday life. In *Language and the politics of emotion,* ed. C. A. Lutz and L. Abu-Lughod, 1–23. Cambridge: Cambridge University Press.

Maatsch, J., and R. Huang. 1986. An evaluation of the construct validity of four alternative theories of clinical competence. In *Proceedings of the 25th annual RIME conference,* 25:69–74. Chicago: AAMC.

MacDonald, T. K., and M. Ross. 1999. Assessing the accuracy of predictions about dating relationships: How and why do lovers' predictions differ from those made by observers? *Personality and Social Psychology Bulletin* 25:1417–1429.

Madsen, C. K., and C. Yarbrough. 1980. *Competency-based music education.* New York: Prentice Hall.

Malone, K., and S. Supri. 2010. A critical time for medical education: The perils of competence-based reform of the curriculum. *Advances in Health Sciences Education.* doi:10.1007/s10459-010-9247-2 http://www.springerlink.com/content/7644146826643605/.

Mann, K. V. 2011. Theoretical perspectives in medical education: Past experience and future possibilities. *Medical Education* 45:60–68.

Mann, K. V., J. Gordon, and A. MacLeod. 2009. Reflection and reflective practice in health professions education: A systematic review. *Advances in Health Sciences Education* 14:595–621.

Mann, K. V., C. P. M. van der Vleuten, K. W. Eva, H. Armson, B. Chesluk, T. Dornan, E. S. Holmboe, J. Lockyer, E. Loney, and J. M Sargeant. 2011. Tensions in informed self-assessment: How the desire for feedback and reticence to collect and use it can conflict. *Academic Medicine* 86:1120–1127.

Marsh, H. W., and L. A. Roche. 1997. Making students' evaluations of teaching effectiveness effective: The critical issues of validity, bias, and utility. *American Psychologist* 52:1187–1197.

McAshan, H. H. 1979. *Competency-based education and behavioral objectives.* Englewood Cliffs, NJ: Educational Technology Publications.

McGaghie, W. C., G. E. Miller, A. Sajid, and T.V. Telder. 1978. *Competency based curriculum development in medical education: An introduction.* Public Health Papers, no. 68. Geneva: World Health Organization.

McIntyre, R. M., and E. Salas. 1995. Measuring and managing for team performance: Emerging principles from complex environments. In *Team effectiveness and decision making in organizations,* ed. R. Guzzo and E. Salas, 149–203. San Francisco: Jossey-Bass.

Medical School Objectives Project (MSOP). 1999. Learning objectives for medical student education: Guidelines for medical schools; Report 1 of the Medical School Objectives Project. *Academic Medicine* 74:13–18.

Meegan, S. P., and C. A. Berg. 2002. Contexts, functions, forms, and processes of collaborative everyday problem solving in older adulthood. *International Journal of Behavioral Development* 26 (1): 6–15.

Meichenbaum, D. 1996. Stress inoculation training for coping with stressors. *Clinical Psychology* 49:4–7.

Messick, S. 1994. The interplay of evidence and consequences in the validation of performance assessments. *Educational Researcher* 23 (2): 13–23.

Meyer, D. E., and D. E. Kieras. 1997a. A computational theory of executive cognitive processes and multiple-task performance, part 1: Basic mechanisms. *Psychological Review* 104 (1): 3–65.

———. 1997b. A computational theory of executive cognitive processes and multiple-task performance, part 2: Accounts of psychological refractory-period phenomena. *Psychological Review* 104 (4): 749–791.

Meyer, D. E., D. E. Kieras, E. Lauber, E. H. Schumacher, J. Glass, E. Zurbriggen, L. Gmeindl, and D. Apfelblat. 1995. Adaptive executive control: Flexible multiple-task performance without pervasive immutable response-selection bottlenecks. *Acta Psychologica* 90 (1–3): 163–190.

Miller, G. 1990. The assessment of clinical skills/competence/performance. *Academic Medicine* 65:S63–S67.

Miller, K. 2007. Compassionate communication in the workplace: Exploring processes of noticing, connecting and responding. *Journal of Applied Communication Research* 35 (3): 223–245.

Miller, R. B. 1978. The information system designer. In *The analysis of practical skills,* ed. W. T. Singleton, 278–291. Baltimore: University Park Press.

Ministry of Education, Ministry of Colleges and Universities. 1980. *Issues and directions: The response of the final report of the Commission on Declining School Enrolments in Ontario.* Toronto: Government of Ontario.

Mittendorf, K., F. Geijsel, A. Howeve, M. de Laat, and L. Nieuwenhuis. 2006. Communities of practice as stimulating forces for collective learning. *Journal of Workplace Learning* 18:298–312.

Monrouxe, L. V. 2010. Identity, identification and medical education: Why should we care? *Medical Education* 44 (1): 40–49.

Montgomery Hunter, K. 1991. *Doctor's stories: The narrative structure of medical knowledge.* Princeton, NJ: Princeton University Press.

Moray, N. 1959. Attention in dichotic-listening: Affective cues and the influence of instructions. *Quarterly Journal of Experimental Psychology* 11 (1): 56–60.

———. 1967. Where is capacity limited? A survey and a model. *Acta Psychologica (Amsterdam)* 27:84–92.

Morris, J. S., B. DeGelder, L. Weiskrantz, and R. J. Dolan. 2001. Modulation of human amygdala activity by emotional learning and conscious awareness. *Nature* 393:467–470.

Moulton, C. A., and R. M. Epstein. 2011. Self-monitoring in surgical practice: Slowing down when you should. *Advances in Medical Education* 2 (part 2): 169–182. doi:10.1007/978–94–007–1682–7_10, http://www.springerlink.com/content/mtv229nnw3302r57/.

Moulton, C. A., G. Regehr, L. Lingard, C. Merritt, and H. MacRae. 2010a. Slowing down to stay out of trouble in the operating room: Remaining attentive in automaticity. *Academic Medicine* 85 (10): 1571–1577.

Moulton, C. A., G. Regehr, L. Lingard, C. Merritt, and H. MacRae. 2010b. "Slowing down when you should": Initiators and influences of the transition from the routine to the effortful. *Journal of Gastrointestinal Surgery* 14 (6): 1019–1026.

Moulton, C. A., G. Regehr, M. Mylopoulos, and H. M. MacRae. 2007. Slowing down when you should: A new model of expert judgment. *Academic Medicine* 82 (10 suppl): S109–S116.

Mylopoulos, M., and G. Regehr. 2007. Cognitive metaphors of expertise and knowledge: Prospects and limitations for medical education. *Medical Education* 41 (12): 1159–1165.

———. 2011. Putting the expert together again. *Medical Education* 45 (9): 920–926.

Mylopoulos, M., and M. Scardamalia. 2008. Doctors' perspectives on their innovations in daily practice: Implications for knowledge building in health care. *Medical Education* 42 (10): 975–981.

Mylopoulos, M., and N. N. Woods. 2009. Having our cake and eating it too: Seeking the best of both worlds in expertise research. *Medical Education* 43 (5): 406–413.

Nabi, R. L. 2003. Exploring the framing effects of emotion: Do discrete emotions differentially influence information accessibility, information seeking, and policy preference? *Communication Research* 30 (2): 224–247.

Naqvi, N., B. Shiv, and A. Bechara. 2006. The role of emotion on decision making. *Current Directions in Psychological Science* 15 (5): 260–264.

Navarro, V. 1999. Health and equity in the world in the era of "globalization." *International Journal of Health Services* 29:215–226.

Neisser, U. 1976. *Cognition and reality: Principles and implications of cognitive psychology.* San Francisco: W. H. Freeman.

Nelson, S., and M. E. Purkis. 2004. Mandatory reflection: The Canadian reconstitution of the competence nurse. *Nursing Inquiry* 11:247–257.

Niedenthal, P. M., and M. B. Setterlund. 1994. Emotion congruence in perception. *Personality and Social Psychology Bulletin* 20 (4): 401–411.

Nisbett, R. E., K. Peng, I. Choi, and A. Norenzayan. 2001. Culture and systems of thought: Holistic versus analytic cognition. *Psychological Review* 108 (2): 291–310.

Nisbett, R. E., and T. D. Wilson. 1977. Telling more than we can know: Verbal reports on mental processes. *Psychological Review* 84 (3): 231–259.

Noddings, N. 1984. *Caring: A feminine approach to ethics and moral education.* Berkeley: University of California Press.

Nonaka, I. 1994. A dynamic theory of organizational knowledge creation. *Organization Science* 5 (1): 14–37.

Nonaka, I., and H. Takeuchi. 1995. *The knowledge-creating company: How Japanese companies create the dynamics of innovation.* New York: Oxford University Press.

Norman, G. R. 1988. Problem-solving skills, solving problems and problem-based learning. *Medical Education* 22:270–286.

———. 2005a. Editorial: Inverting the pyramid. *Advances in Health Sciences Education Theory and Practice* 10:85–88.

———. 2005b. Research in clinical reasoning: Past history and current trends. *Medical Education* 39 (4): 418–427.

———. 2006. Editorial: Outcomes, objectives, and the seductive appeal of simple solutions. *Advances in Health Science Education: Theory and Practice* 11:217–220.

———. 2009. Teaching basic science to optimize transfer. *Medical Teacher* 31 (9): 807–811.

Norman, G. R., and L. R. Brooks. 1997. The non-analytical basis of clinical reasoning. *Advances in Health Science Education* 2 (2): 173–184.

Norman, G. R., E. K. M. Smith, A. C. Powles, P. J. Rooney, N. L. Henry, and P. E. Dodd. 1987. Factors underlying performance on written tests of knowledge. *Medical Education* 21:297–304.

Norman, G. R., D. Swanson, and S. M. Case. 1996. Conceptual and methodology issues in studies comparing assessment formats, issues in comparing item formats. *Teaching and Learning in Medicine* 8 (4): 208–216.

Norton, S. A., and B. J. Bowers. 2001. Working toward consensus: Providers' strategies to shift patients from curative to palliative treatment choices. *Research in Nursing & Health* 24 (4): 258–269.

Nussbaum, M. 1996. Compassion: The basic social emotion. *Social Philosophy and Policy* 13 (1): 27–58.

Nussbaum A. D., and C. S. Dweck. 2008. Defensiveness versus remediation: Self-theories and modes of self-esteem maintenance. *Personality and Social Psychology Bulletin* 34:599–612.

Oandasan, I., D. D'Amour, M. Zwarenstein, K. Barker, M. Purden, M. Beaulieu, S. Reeves, L. Nasmith, C. Bosco, L. Ginsburg, and D. Tregunno. 2004. *Interdisciplinary education for collaborative, patient-centred practice.* Ottawa: Health Canada.

Oandasan, I., and S. Reeves. 2005. Key elements for interprofessional education, part 1: The learner, the educator and the learning context. *Journal of Interprofessional Care* 19:21–38.

Ochsner, K. N., S. A. Bunge, J. J. Gross, and J. D. Gabrieli. 2002. Rethinking feelings: An fMRI study of the cognitive regulation of emotion. *Journal of Cognitive Neuroscience* 14:1215–1229.

Ogawa, T., and H. Komatsu. 2004. Target selection in area V4 during a multidimensional visual search task. *Journal of Neuroscience* 24 (28): 6371–6382.

Orlander, J. D., T. W. Barber, and B. G. Fincke. 2002. The morbidity and mortality conference: The delicate nature of learning from error. *Academic Medicine* 77 (10): 1001–1006.

Paavola, S., L. Lipponen, and K. Hakkarainen. 2004. Models of innovative knowledge communities and three metaphors of learning. *Review of Educational Research* 74 (4): 557–577.

Palmer, P. J. 2007. *The courage to teach: Exploring the inner landscape of a teacher's life.* 10th anniversary ed. San Francisco: Jossey-Bass.

Parry J., J. Mathers, A. Stevens, A. Parsons, R. Lilford, P. Spurgeon, and H. Thomas. 2006. Admissions processes for five year medical courses at English schools: Review. *British Medical Journal* 332:1005. doi:10.1136/bmj.38768.590174.55.

Patterson, F., E. Ferguson, P. Lane, K. Farrell, J. Martlew, and A. Wells. 2000. A competency model for general practice: Implications for selection, training, and development. *British Journal of General Practice* 50:188–193.

Pea, R. D. 1993. Practice of distributed intelligence and designs for education. In *Distributed cognitions: Psychological and educational considerations,* ed. G. Salomon, 47–87. New York: Cambridge University Press.

Peck, C., M. McCall, B. McLaren, and T. Rotem. 2000. Continuing medical education and continuing professional development: International comparisons. *British Medical Journal* 320:432–435.

Pessoa, L. 2008. On the relationship between emotion and cognition. *Nature Reviews Neuroscience* 9 (2): 148–158.

Peters, E., J. Hibbard, P. Slovic, and N. Dieckmann. 2007. Numeracy skill and the communication, comprehension, and use of risk-benefit information. *Health Affairs* 26 (3): 741–748.

Pfeifer, J. H., and M. Dapretto. 2009. Mirror, mirror, in my mind: Empathy, interpersonal competence, and the mirror neuron system. In *The social neuroscience of empathy,* ed. J. Decety and W. Ickes, 183–197: Cambridge, MA: MIT Press.

Phelps, E. A. 2006. Emotion and cognition: Insights from studies on the human amygdala. *Annual Review of Psychology* 57:27–53.

Pickett, C. E. 1857. *Oration delivered in the Congregational Church, Sacramento, California, July 4, 1857.* San Francisco: Whitten, Towne and Excelsior Steam Presses.

Plass, J. L., R. Moreno, and R. Brünken. 2010. *Cognitive load theory.* New York: Cambridge University Press.

Polanyi, M. 2003. *Personal knowledge towards a post-critical philosophy.* London: Routledge.

Pontecorvo, C. 1993. Developing literacy skills through cooperative computer use: Issues for learning and instruction. In *Designing environments for constructive learning,* ed. T. Duffy, J. Lowyck, and D. Jonassen, 139–160. New York: Springer-Verlag.

Popham, W. J., and T. R. Husek. 1969. Implications of criterion-referenced measurement. *Journal of Educational Measurement* 6 (1): 1–9.

Pronin, E., D. Y. Lin, and L. Ross. 2002. The bias blind spot: Perceptions of bias in self versus others. *Personality and Social Psychology Bulletin* 28:369–381.

Pronovost, P., S. Berenholtz, T. Dorman, P. A. Lipsett, T. Simmonds, and C. Haraden. 2003. Improving communication in the ICU using daily goals. *Journal of Critical Care* 18:71–75.

Pugh, M. 2005. Maintenance of certification for family physicians from the American Board of Family Medicine. *Annals of Family Medicine* 3:91–92.

Rabow, M., R. Reman, D. Parmelee, and T. Innui. 2010. Professional formation: Extending medicine's lineage of service into the next century. *Academic Medicine* 85 (2): 310–317.

Raghunathan, R., and M. T. Pham. 1999. All negative moods are not equal: Motivational influences of anxiety and sadness on decision making. *Organizational Behavior and Human Decision Processes* 79 (1): 56–77.

Reeves, S., A. Fox, and B. D. Hodges. 2009. The competency movement in the health professions: Ensuring consistent standards or reproducing conventional domains of practice? *Advances in Health Sciences Education* 14:451–453.

Reeves, S., M. Zwarenstein, J. Goldman, H. Barr, D. Freeth, M. Hammick, and I. Koppel. 2008. Interprofessional education: Effects on professional practice and health care outcomes. *Cochrane Database of Systematic Reviews* 23 (1): CD002213.

Regehr, C., V. R. LeBlanc, R. B. Jelley, and I. Barath. 2008. Acute stress and performance in police recruits. *Stress and Health* 24 (4): 295–303.

Regehr, G., and K. W. Eva. 2006. Self-assessment, self-direction, and the self-regulating professional. *Clinical Orthopaedics and Related Research* 449:34–38.

Regehr, G., and M. Mylopoulos. 2008. Maintaining competence in the field: Learning about practice, through practice, in practice. *Journal of Continuing Education in the Health Professions* 28:S19–S23.

Regehr, G., and G. F. Norman. 1996. Issues in cognitive psychology: Implications for professional education. *Academic Medicine* 71:988–1001.

Regenbogen, S. E., C. C. Greenberg, D. M. Studdert, S. R. Lipsitz, M. J. Zinner, and A. A. Gawande. 2007. Patterns of technical error among surgical malpractice claims: An analysis of strategies to prevent injury to surgical patients. *Annals of Surgery* 246 (5): 705–711.

Remington, R. W., J. C. Johnston, and S. Yantis. 1992. Involuntary attentional capture by abrupt onsets. *Perception & Psychophysics* 51 (3): 279–290.

Reyna, V. F., and F. J. Lloyd. 2006. Physician decision making and cardiac risk: Effects of knowledge, risk perception, risk tolerance, and fuzzy processing. *Journal of Experimental Psychology: Applied* 12 (3): 179–195.

Richards, A., C. C. French, A. J. Calder, B. Webb, R. Fox, and A. W. Young. 2002. Anxiety-related bias in the classification of emotionally ambiguous facial expressions. *Emotion* 2 (3): 273–287.

Risucci, D. A., A. J. Tortolani, and R. J. Ward. 1989. Ratings of surgical residents by self, supervisors and peers. *Surgery, Gynecology, and Obstetrics* 169:519–526.

Rizzolatti, G., and L. Craighero. 2004. The mirror-neuron system. *Annual Review of Neuroscience* 27:169–192.

Rogers, E. 1995. *Diffusion of innovations.* New York: The Free Press.

Rogers, R., E. Malancharuvil-Berkes, M. Mosley, D. Hui, and G. O'Garro Joseph. 2005. Critical discourse analysis in education: A review of the literature. *Review of Educational Research* 75:365–416.

Rogoff, B. 1998. Cognition as a collaborative process. In *Handbook of child psychology,* ed. B. Damon, 679–744. New York: Wiley.

Rogoff, B., J. Mistry, A. Goncu, and C. Mosier. 1993. Guided participation in cultural activity by toddlers and caregivers. *Monographs of the Society for Research in Child Development* 58 (8): v–vi, 1–174, discussion 175–179.

Romanow, R. J. 2002. *Building on values: The future of health care in Canada.* Final Report 1–356. Ottawa: Commission on the Future of Health Care in Canada.

Rose, N. 1985. *The psychological complex: Psychology, politics and society in England, 1869–1939.* London: Routledge.

Royal College of Physicians and Surgeons of Canada (RCPSC). 2007. Maintenance of certification program. http://rcpsc.medical.org/opa/moc-program/index.php (accessed July 5, 2011).

Rubin, N. J., M. Bebeau, I. W. Leigh, J. W. Lichtenberg, P. D. Nelson, S. Portnoy, I. L. Smith, and N. J. Kaslow. 2007. The competency movement within psychology: An historical perspective. *Professional Psychology: Research and Practice* 38:452–462.

Rusbult, C. E., E. J. Finkel, and M. Kumashiro. 2009. The Michelangelo phenomenon. *Current Directions in Psychological Science* 18:305–309.

Salas, E., C. Prince, D. P. Baker, and L. Shrestha. 1995. Situation awareness in team performance: Implications for measurement and training. *Human Factors: The Journal of the Human Factors and Ergonomics Society* 37:123–136.

Salas, E., M. A. Rosen, C. S. Burke, D. Nicholson, and W. R. Howse. 2007. Markers for enhancing team cognition in complex environments: The power of team performance diagnosis. *Aviation, Space, and Environmental Medicine* 78:B77–B85.

Salmon, P. M. 2009. *Distributed situation awareness: Theory, measurement and application to teamwork.* Farnham, Surrey: Ashgate.

Samuels, J. G., and S. J. Fetzer. 2009. Evidence-based pain management: Analyzing the practice environment and clinical expertise. *Clinical Nurse Specialist* 23 (5): 245–251.

Sargeant, J. M., H. Armson, B. Chesluk, T. Dornan, K. W. Eva, E. S. Holmboe, J. Lockyer, E. Loney, K. V. Mann, and C. P. M. van der Vleuten. 2010. The processes and dimensions of informed self-assessment. *Academic Medicine* 85:1212–1220.

Sargeant, J. M., K. V. Mann, S. N. Ferrier, D. B. Langille, P. D. Muirhead, V. M. Hayes, and D. E. Sinclair. 2003. Responses of rural family physicians and their colleague and coworker raters to a multi-source feedback process: A pilot study. *Academic Medicine* 78:S42–S44.

Satterfield, J., and E. Hughes. 2007. Emotion skills training for medical students: A systematic review. *Medical Education* 41:935–941.

Satterwhite, R. C., W. M. Satterwhite, and C. Enarson. 2000. An ethical paradox: The effect of unethical conduct on medical students' values. *Journal of Medical Ethics* 26:462–465.

Saunders, T., J. E. Driskell, J. H. Johnston, and E. Salas. 1996. The effects of stress inoculation training on anxiety and performance. *Journal of Occupational and Health Psychology* 1 (2): 170–186.

Scardamalia, M. 2004. Computer supported intentional learning environments/knowledge forum. In *Education and Technology: An encyclopedia,* ed. A. Kovalchick and K. Dawson, 183–192. Santa Barbara: ABC-CLIO.

Scardamalia, M., and C. Bereiter. 2003a. Knowledge building. In *Encyclopedia of education,* ed. J. Guthrie, 1370–1373. New York: Macmillan Reference

———. 2003b. Knowledge building environments: Extending the limits of the possible in education and knowledge work. In *Encyclopedia of distributed learning,* ed. A. DiStefano, K. E. Rudestam, and R. Silverman, 269–272. Thousand Oaks, CA: Sage.

Scheele, F., P. Teunissen, S. Van Luijk, E. Heineman, L. Fluit, H. Mulder, A. Meininger, et al. 2008. Introducing competency-based postgraduate medical education in the Netherlands. *Medical Teacher* 30:248–253.

Schmeichel, B. J., and R. F. Baumeister. 2010. Effortful attention control. In *Effortless attention: A new perspective in the cognitive science of attention and action,* ed. B. Bruya, 24–49. Cambridge, MA: MIT Press.

Schmidt, H., and H. P. Boshuizen. 1993. On acquiring expertise in medicine. *Educational Psychology Review* 5 (3): 205–221.

Schmidt, H. G., G. R. Norman, and H. P. Boshuizen. 1990. A cognitive perspective on medical expertise: Theory and implication. *Academic Medicine* 65 (10): 611–621.

Schmidt, R. A. 1991. Frequent augmented feedback can degrade learning: Evidence and interpretations. In *Tutorials in motor neuroscience,* ed. G. E. Stelmach and J. Requin, 59–75. Dordrecht: Kluwer.

Schön, D. 1983. *The reflective practitioner: How professionals think in action.* London: Temple Smith.

———. 1987. *Educating the reflective practitioner: Toward a new design for teaching and learning in the professions.* San Francisco: Jossey-Bass.

Schuwirth, L. W. T., L. Southgate, G. Page, N. Paget, J. Lescop, S. Lew, and W. Wade. 2002. When enough is enough: Testing a model for the assessment of performance in clinical practice. Paper presented at the 10th Ottawa Conference on Medical Education, July 13–16, Ottawa.

Schuwirth, L. W. T., and C. P. M. van der Vleuten. 2006. A plea for new psychometric models in educational assessment. *Medical Education* 40:296–300.

Schwartz, D. L., and J. D. Bransford. 1998. A time for telling. *Cognition and Instruction* 16 (4): 475–523.

Schwartz, D. L., J. D. Bransford, and D. Sears. 2005. Efficiency and innovation in transfer. In *Transfer of learning for a modern multidisciplinary perspective,* ed. J. Mestre, 1–51. Greenwich, CT: Information Age.

Segouin, C., and B. D. Hodges. 2005. Educating physicians in France and Canada: Are the differences based on evidence or history? *Medical Education* 39:1205–1212.

Segouin, C., B. D. Hodges, and P. H. Brechat. 2005. Globalization in health care: Is international standardization of quality a step toward outsourcing? *International Journal for Quality in Health Care* 17:277–279.

Sfard, A. 1998. On two metaphors for learning and the dangers of choosing just one. *Education Research* 27:4–13.

Shanafelt, T. D., C. M. Balch, G. Bechamps, T. Russell, L. Dyrbye, D. Satele, P. Collicott, P. J. Novotny, J. Sloan, and J. Freischlag. 2010. Burnout and medical errors among American surgeons. *Annals of Surgery* 251 (6): 995–1000.

Sherbino, J., J. R. Frank, L. Flynn, and L. Snell. 2011. "Intrinsic roles" rather than "armour": Renaming the "non-medical expert roles" of the CanMEDS framework to match their intent. *Advances in Health Science Education: Theory and Practice* 16:695–697.

Shorter, E. 1985. *Doctors and their patients: A social history.* New York: Simon & Schuster.

Shute, V. J. 2008. Focus on formative feedback. *Review of Educational Research* 78:153–189.

Sidhom, M. A., and M. G. Poulsen. 2006. Multidisciplinary care in oncology: Medicolegal implications of group decisions. *Lancet Oncology* 7:951–954.

Siegel, D. J. 2007. *The mindful brain: Reflection and attunement in the cultivation of well-being.* New York: W. W. Norton.

Simons, D. J. 2000. Attentional capture and inattentional blindness. *Trends in Cognitive Sciences* 4 (4): 147–155.

Simpson, J. G., J. Furnace, J. Crosby, A. D. Cumming, P. A. Evans, B. Friedman, M. David, et al. 2002. The Scottish doctor: Learning outcomes for the medical undergraduate in Scotland; A foundation for competent and reflective practitioners. *Medical Teacher* 24:136–143.

Sinclair, L., M. Lowe, T. Paulenko, and A. Walczak. 2007. *Facilitating interprofessional clinical learning: Interprofessional education placements and other opportunities.* Toronto: University of Toronto, Office of Interprofessional Education.

Skemp, R. R. 1979. *Intelligence, learning, and action: A foundation for theory and practice in education.* Chichester: Wiley.

Skinner, B. 1953. *Science and human behavior.* New York: Simon & Schuster.

Social Sciences and Humanities Council of Canada (SSHRC). 2009. Applying for funding: Definition of applicant. http://www.sshrc-crsh.gc.ca/site/apply-demande/background-renseignements/definitions-eng.aspx#a1 (accessed January 28, 2010).

Solomon, R. C. 2007. *True to our feelings: What our emotions are telling us.* Oxford: Oxford Universty Press. Spafford, M. M., C. F. Schryer, and L. Lingard. 2008. The rhetoric of patient voice: Reported talk with patients in referral and consultation letters. *Communication and Medicine* 5:183–194.

Spencer H. 1862. *First Principles.* London: Williams and Norgate.

Spencer, J. 2004. Decline in empathy in medical education: How can we stop the rot? *Medical Education* 38 (9): 916–918.

Starr, P. 1982. *The social transformation of American medicine: The rise of a sovereign profession and the making of a vast industry.* New York: Basic Books.

Stern D. T., A. Wojtczak, and R. Schwarz. 2006. The assessment of global minimum essential requirements in medical education. Institute for International Medical Education. http://www.iime.org/documents/assessment.htm (accessed December 3, 2011).

Strong-Boag, V. J. 1981. Canada's women doctors: Feminism constrained. In *Medicine in Canadian society: Historical perspectives,* ed. S. E. D. Shortt, 109–129. Montreal: McGill-Queen's University Press.

Student Doctor Network Forum. (2010) Posted online reply from one physician (Sergio 99) to another's (Bobblehead) discussion thread. http://forums.studentdoctor.net/showthread.php?p = 9282617 (accessed March 5, 2010).

Suchman, A. L., and D. A. Matthews. 1988. What makes the patient-doctor relationship therapeutic? Exploring the connexional dimension of medical care. *Annals of Internal Medicine* 108 (1): 125–130.

Sullivan, W. 2011. Preparing professionals as moral agents. Carnegie Foundation for the Advancement of Teaching. http://www.carnegiefoundation.org/perspectives/preparing-professionals-moral-agents (accessed December 8, 2011).

Sveiby, K. E. 1997. *The new organizational wealth: Managing and measuring knowledge based assets.* San Francisco: Berrett Koehler.

Swaminathan, H., R. K. Hambleton, and J. Algina. 1974. Reliability of criterion-referenced tests: A decision-theoretic formulation. *Journal of Educational Measurement* 11 (4): 263–267.

Talbot, M. 2004. Monkey see, monkey do: A critique of the competency model in graduate medical education. *Medical Education* 38:587–592.

Tavris, C., and E. Aronson. 2007. *Mistakes were made (but not by me): Why we justify foolish beliefs, bad decisions, and hurtful acts.* New York: Harcourt.

Taylor, F. W. 1911. *Principles of scientific management.* New York: Harper.

Taylor, J. S. 2003. Confronting "culture" in medicine's "culture of no culture." *Academic Medicine* 78:555–559.

Teeple, G. 2000. *Globalization and the decline of social reform: Into the twenty-first century.* Amherst, NY: Humanity Books.

ten Cate, O. 2005. Entrustability of professional activities and competency-based training. *Medical Education* 39:1176–1177.

Theeuwes, J. 1992. Perceptual selectivity for color and form. *Perception & Psychophysics* 51 (6): 599–606.

Thorndike, E. L. 1922. Measurement in education. In *Intelligence tests and their uses,* ed. G. Montrose Whipple, 1–9. Bloomington, IL: National Society for the Study of Education, Public School Publishing.

Thorndike, E. L., and R. S. Woodworth. 1901. The influence of improvement in one mental function upon the efficiency of other functions. *Psychological Review* 8:247–261.

Toft, B., and P. Gooderham. 2009. Involuntary automaticity: A potential legal defence against an allegation of clinical negligence? *Quality & Safety in Health Care* 18 (1): 69–73.

Tragically Hip. 1992. At the hundredth meridian. http://en.wikipedia.org/wiki/At_the_Hundredth_Meridian (accessed November 28, 2011).

Treisman, A. 2006. How the deployment of attention determines what we see. *Visual Cognition* 14 (4–8): 411–443.

Tversky, A., and D. Kahneman. 1973. Availability: A heuristic for judging frequency and probability. *Cognitive Psychology* 5:207–232.

Vallone, R. P., D. W. Griffin, S. Lin, and L. Ross. 1990. Overconfident prediction of future actions and outcomes by self and others. *Journal of Personality and Social Psychology* 58:582–592.

Van der Vleuten, C. P. M., G. R. Norman, and E. De Graaf. 1991. Pitfalls in the pursuit of objectivity: Issues of reliability. *Medical Education* 25:110–118.

van de Wiel, M. W. J., H. P. A. Boshuizen, and H. G. Schmidt. 2000. Knowledge restructuring in expertise development: Evidence from pathophysiological representations of clinical cases by students and physicians. *European Journal of Cognitive Psychology* 12 (3): 323–355.

Van Merriënboer, J. J. G., and J. Sweller. 2005. Cognitive load theory and complex learning: Recent developments and future directions. *Educational Psychology Review* 17 (2): 147–177.

——. 2010. Cognitive load theory in health professional education: Design principles and strategies. *Medical Education* 44 (1): 85–93.

Varpio, L., C. F. Schryer, and L. Lingard. 2009. Routine and adaptive expert strategies for resolving ICT mediated communication problems in the team setting. *Medical Education* 43 (7): 680–687.

Voyer, S., and D. Pratt. 2011. Feedback: Much more than a tool. *Medical Education* 45:862–864.

Vygotsky, L. S. 1978. *Mind in society: The development of higher psychological processes.* Cambridge, MA: Harvard University Press.

Wallace, P. 1997. Following the treads of innovation: The history of standardized patients in medical education. *Caduceus* 13:5–28.

Walton, M. D., and S. L. Elliot. 2006. Improving safety and quality: How can education help? *Medical Journal of Australia* 184:S60–S64.

Ward, M., L. D. Gruppen, and G. Regehr. 2001. Research in self-assessment: Current state of the art. *Advances in Health Sciences Education* 7:63–80.

Watling, C. J., C. Kenyon, E. Zibrowski, V. Shulz, M. Goldszmidt, I. Singh, H. Maddocks, and L. Lingard. 2008. Rules of engagement: Residents' perceptions of the in-training evaluation process. *Academic Medicine* 83:S97–S100.

Wear, D. 2008. On outcomes and humility. *Academic Medicine* 83:625–626.

Weaver, R. 1953. *The ethics of rhetoric.* South Bend, IN: Henry Regenery.

Weick, K. E. 1995. *Sensemaking in organizations.* Thousand Oaks, CA: Sage.

Weick, K. E., and K. M. Sutcliffe. 2001. *Managing the unexpected: Assuring high performance in an age of complexity.* University of Michigan Business School Management Series. San Francisco: Jossey-Bass.

Weick, K. E., K. M. Sutcliffe, and D. Obstfeld. 2005. Organizing and the process of sensemaking. *Organization Science* 16 (4): 409–421.

Wellens, A. R. 1993. Group situation awareness and distributed decision making: From military to civilian applications. In *Individual and group decision making: Current issues,* ed. N. J. Castellan, 267–291. Hillsdale, NJ: Erlbaum.

Wenger, E. 1998. *Communities of practice: Learning, meaning, and identity.* Cambridge: Cambridge University Press.

Wetzel, C. M., S. A. Black, G. B. Hanna, T. Athanasiou, R. L. Kneebone, D. Nestel, J. H. N. Wolfe, and M. Woloshynowych. 2010. The effects of stress and coping on surgical performance during simulations. *Annals of Surgery* 251 (1): 171–176.

Whalen, P. J., S. L. Rauch, N. L. Etcoff, S. C. McInerney, M. B. Lee, and M. A. Jenike. 1998. Masked presentations of emotional facial expressions modulate amygdala activity without explicit knowledge. *Journal of Neuroscience* 18 (1): 411–418.

Whitehead, C. R., Z. Austin, and B. D. Hodges. 2011. Flower power: The armoured expert in the CanMEDS competency framework? *Advances in Health Science Education: Theory and Practice* 16:681–694.

Williams, S. 2001. *Emotion and social theory.* London. Sage.

Witz, A. 1992. *Professions and patriarchy.* London: Macmillan.

Zaini, R. G., K. A. Bin Abdulrahman, A. A. Al-Khotani, A. M. A. Al-Hayani, I. A. Al-Alwan, and S. D. Jastaniah. 2011. Saudi meds: A competence specification for Saudi medical graduates. *Medical Teacher* 33:582–584.

Zeelenberg, M., K. van der Bos, E. van Dijk, and R. Pieters. 2002. The inaction effect in the psychology of regret. *Journal of Personality and Social Psychology* 82 (3): 314–327.

Contributors

Ronald M. Epstein, MD, professor, Department of Family Medicine, director of the Center for Communication and Disparities Research and director of the Deans Teaching Fellowship Program at the University of Rochester. Ron is a family physician, medical educator, and researcher who is widely recognized for his influential publications on communication, mindfulness and reflection in health care, and frameworks for understanding and assessing physician competence.

Kevin W. Eva, PhD, associate professor, senior scientist, Centre for Health Education Scholarship, University of British Columbia; editor in chief, *Medical Education*. Kevin is a cognitive psychologist whose leadership at the top journal of medical education and research on the nature of competence, self-assessment, and judgment is pushing the field in important ways.

Larry D. Gruppen, PhD, professor and chair, Department of Medical Education, University of Michigan Medical School. Larry is one of the United

States' leading researchers in medical education and holds an endowed chair as the Josiah Macy Jr. Professor of Medical Education. His work focuses on clinical expertise development, competency definition and assessment, and educational research development.

Brian D. Hodges, MD, PhD, FRCPC, professor and scientist, Wilson Centre for Research in Education; Richard and Elizabeth Currie Chair in Health Professions Education Research, Faculty of Medicine, University of Toronto; and vice president, education, University Health Network (Toronto General, Toronto Western, and Princess Margaret hospitals). Brian is a psychiatrist, medical educator, and former director of one of the largest centers for medical education research in the world. His research, writing, and presentations push the boundaries of what it is possible to think and say about the concept of competence.

Vicki LeBlanc, PhD, assistant professor, Faculty of Dentistry; scientist, Wilson Centre for Research in Education, University of Toronto. A graduate of McMaster University, Vicki is a cognitive psychologist whose research and leadership in simulation and the role of stress in clinical competence has altered understanding and practice in medical and allied health professions.

Annie S. O. Leung, BASc, senior medical student, Wilson Centre for Research in Education, University of Toronto. Blending her engineering background with interests in psychology and sociology, Annie has explored competence in the context of surgical decision making and surgical error under the guidance of Dr. Carol-Anne Moulton.

Lorelei Lingard, PhD, professor, Department of Medicine, University of Western Ontario (Western); inaugural director of the Centre for Education Research & Innovation at the Schulich School of Medicine & Dentistry at Western. One of medical education's most widely published and cited researchers, Lorelei's work on team communication and patient safety has revolutionized thinking and practice in health care delivery and education research.

Nancy McNaughton MEd, PhD, associate director, Standardized Patient Program, University of Toronto. Nancy is a researcher and scholar in the field of simulation and standardized patients, known particularly for her innovative work on discourses of emotion and technologies of simulation.

Carol-Anne E. Moulton, MBBS, MEd, PhD, assistant professor, Department of Surgery; scientist, Wilson Centre, University of Toronto. Carol-Anne is a hepatobiliary surgeon who completed doctoral studies in medical education and is now conducting innovative research on competence in the operating room.

Maria Mylopoulos, PhD, assistant professor, Department of Pediatrics, cross-appointed scientist, Wilson Centre, University of Toronto; education researcher, Sick Kids Learning Institute. Maria is a graduate of doctoral studies in education, bringing to health professional education a critical look at the intersections of expertise, innovation, and specialization.

Glenn Regehr PhD, professor, Department of Surgery, and associate director, research, Centre for Health Education Scholarship, Faculty of Medicine, University of British Columbia. A leader of health professional education research methodology for over two decades, Glenn is an influential figure in shaping and advancing the quality of research and critiquing its inconsistencies and challenges. He conducts groundbreaking work on self-assessment and assessment of competence.

Lambert W. T. Schuwirth, PhD, strategic professor, Flinders Innovation in Clinical Education, Flinders University, Adelaide, Australia and professor, Faculty of Medicine, University of Maastricht, Netherlands. Lambert is a prolific writer and researcher in the field of education and assessment of competence, and an original thinker and critic in the area of the psychometric paradigm.

Cees P. M. van der Vleuten, PhD, professor of Education, chair, Department of Educational Development and Research; scientific director, School of Health Professions Education, Faculty of Health, Medicine and Life Sciences, Maastricht University, Netherlands. Cees has been a leader of both medical education practice and research for over three decades, one of the world's most-respected and cited figures in this area. Bringing fresh critical thinking to the field of competence, he continues to push the limits of assessment practices and integrate new perspectives.

INDEX

Note: Italic page numbers refer to tables.

MainCert, 52
maintenance of competence (MOC): and
    individualist discourse of competence,
    52–53; and self-assessment, 132
malpractice claims, 53
Mann, K. V., 145, 149
Marsh, H. W., 150
McGaghie, W. C., 68
McGuire, D., 50
McMaster University, 35
McNaughton, Nancy, 10, 167, 172
medical competence: construction of,
    18; discourses of, 9; and emotional
    competence, 10; global definition of,
    7; image of, 17–18, 19; and shifting
    cultural expectations, 18–19; and
    team-based practice, 9–10, 43
medical education: behaviorism in,
    26; and character formation, 88;
    competency-based curriculum in,
    2, 3–5; and emotional intelligence,
    85; and faculty development, 41;
    and global economy, 4, 7–8, 36;
    and individualist discourse of
    competence, 46–47, 49–50, 53–54;
    international partnerships in, 3, 4;
    and knowledge discourse, 33, 37, 38,
    41, 47; and performance discourse,
    33, 34, 35, 37, 41, 47; and production
    discourse, 31, 32, 34, 36, 37, 41, 47;
    and psychometric discourse, 27,
    33, 34, 35–36, 37, 41; and reflection
    discourse, 30, 33, 34, 37, 41, 47; role
    of basic science in, 40. *See also* health
    professional education; medical
    school admissions
medical licensure examinations,
    physician competencies on, 16
medical practice: and competency-
    based curriculum, 2; construction
    of, 18; and emotional regulation, 87;
    so-called "soft" aspects of, 35, 114;
    and uncertainty, 12. *See also* health
    professional practice; team-based
    practice

medical school admissions: candidate-
    selection strategy in, 4; and
    discourse of competence, 41; and
    emotional intelligence, 85; and
    emotions, 94–95; and psychometric
    discourse, 29
Medical School Objectives Project
    (MSOP), 44
Meehl, P. E., 117
memory: and emotions, 71, 73, 77, 80,
    81, 82, 83, 94; and executive attention,
    169; and intuition, 167; and self-
    assessment, 141, 145, 151–152
Messick, S., 117
metacognition: and automaticity,
    165–166, 167; and mindfulness,
    164–166, 175
Miller, George, 25, 26
Miller, K., 91
mindfulness: habits of mindful practice,
    167–169; and metacognition, 164–166,
    175; and reflection discourse, 30; and
    self-monitoring, 156; and shared
    mind, 173–175; as skill, 176; and
    slowing-down moments, 12, 168; and
    sociocultural pressures, 173
Mittendorf, K., 56
Mooney, C. J., 68–69
Moore, J. L., 110
Moulton, Carol-Anne, 12, 80, 82, 93
multidimensional thinking, 41
mutual performance monitoring, 60
Mylopoulos, Maria, 10

negative transfer of learning, 110
Neisser, U., 164
Nelson, S., 31, 37
neuroscience perspective, and emotions,
    10, 74–75, 76, 77–80, 83, 94, 95, 167
Nonaka, I., 58
Norman, G. R., 26–27, 152

objective assessment: as "god term," 44;
    and medical education, 1
objective scientific fact, and emotions, 70